How I Found Meaning
Widowhood, Firehouses, & Organic Vegetables

"Every now and then a book comes along that deeply touches your heart. Not only is *How I Found Meaning (And Humor) in Widowhood, Firehouses, & Organic Vegetables* a must-read for anyone who's experienced a loss, it's also an inspirational road map for how to discover renewed meaning and purpose, and how to take charge of your health through the power of Functional Medicine."

—Sandra Scheinbaum, Founder and CEO, Functional Medicine Coaching Academy

"Marie is a masterful storyteller. Her ability to walk the reader through the trenches of grief and her own discovery of new purpose is the perfect road map for anyone who has lost a loved one. What I love most is her ability to find humor and love tucked in the grieving process. Life is messy and beautiful, and she perfectly captures that. That is what we should all search for . . . her ability to take tragedy and create meaningful, powerful purpose for our lives. This is a must-read for grievers and non-grievers alike."

—Whitney McDuff, Speaker Brand Strategist, Speaker PR, Author

"There's no denying it: loss touches all. Exceptional and extraordinary people turn personal loss into precious gifts for the lives of others. True to the marvelous Marie Scott's indomitable spirit, *How I Found Meaning (And Humor) in Widowhood, Firehouses, & Organic Vegetables: 7 Steps to Healing After Loss* is a gift that keeps giving. Marie's book allows vicarious experiences to become inspiring catalysts for meaning, purpose, laughter, and love to flourish again, as well as guiding the reader to healing through functional medicine practices."

—Mahnaz Malik, FMCHC, NBC-HWC

"How I Found Meaning (and Humor) in Widowhood, Firehouses & Organic Vegetables is a story of hope and transformation. Marie teaches us how life is meant to be embraced every step of the way in our relationships with those closest to us and through our relationship with self and food. Marie honors the first love of her life so beautifully, teaching us how to grieve in a way that is healthy and transformative, and how romantic love can happen once again. This book is a gift."

> —Stacey Crew, Certified Health Coach, and Author of *Mind Body Kitchen: Transform You & Your Kitchen for a Healthier Lifestyle*

"I am honored to be a part of Marie's story, and I know that her spectacularly positive outlook and amazing life transformation will provide many people with hope. By reading this book, you will clearly see how Marie's positive attitude and gratitude played a major role in creating a healthy life, and allowed her to share her message!"

> —Dr. Navaz Habib, Functional Medicine Practitioner, Author of *Activate Your Vagus Nerve: Unleash your body's natural ability to heal*, Founder of Health Upgraded

"Marie Scott hooked me from the beginning through her tender storytelling of love, grief, and rebirth after the tragic loss of her beloved Dave. Marie's *7-Steps to Healing After Loss* is a perfect recipe to restore one's mind, body, and soul to a healthy state of being. She reminds us in a gentle way that life is not just about oneself but also about the people's lives you cast a shadow on during your lifetime."

> —Dr. Troy Hall, Bestselling Author of *Cohesion Culture: Proven Principles to Retain Your Top Talent*, and *FANNY RULES: A Mother's Leadership Lessons That Never Grow Old*

"This practical and insightful book speaks to the needs of a major portion of our population. Whole, healthy, and content again without my mate? Impossible! If death has left you thinking these words, curl up with this book as Marie inspires you to embrace a hopeful vision for the future."

—Dr. Ja'net Bishop Nesbit, EdD, Coach, Speaker, Veteran, Author of *From Grief to Growth: 8 Dimensions to Wellness Through Self-Care, 90-Day Gratitude Journal,* and *How Much Joy Is in Your Journey*

"Marie Scott has brought her story of love, loss, and loving again to us in a way that can help widows and widowers grieve and move on to embrace a healthy lifestyle as they continue through life. She brings her *7 Steps to Healing* to readers, helping them transform heartbreak into a healthy way to move forward after a devastating loss. Her stories are full of hope, honoring the deceased, and guidance to life after loss."

—Lisa Burbage, Workplace Wellness Expert

"I love your book! I have always thought the world of you and Dave but realize, even at that, you and Dave were like this little iceberg—I only knew a portion of you. The full you is even better. As I read your love story, I feel my love story with Candy. It's different, but it has that depth. It is also nice to get your nutritional wisdom through the *7 Steps to Healing.* Good stuff. Or in the words of my son, #goodsoup."

—Lee Barnes, MBA, PMP, Author of *Rings of Deception: Randy Barnes, Drugs, and the Education of an Olympic Champion*

"How I Found Meaning (and Humor) In Widowhood, Firehouses, & Organic Vegetables: 7 Steps to Healing After Loss is a lively, detailed account of love interrupted when her firefighter husband is diagnosed with cancer. Author Marie Scott speaks frankly with energy, attitude, and a professional eye on wellness techniques."

—B. Lynn Goodwin, Author of *Never Too Late: From Wannabe to Wife at 62* and *Talent*

How I Found Meaning (and Humor)
In Widowhood, Firehouses, & Organic Vegetables

by Marie Scott

ISBN 978-1-64663-553-5

Published by

◀ köehlerbooks™

3705 Shore Drive
Virginia Beach, VA 23455
800-435-4811
www.koehlerbooks.com

HOW I FOUND MEANING

(and Humor)

IN WIDOWHOOD, FIREHOUSES, & ORGANIC VEGETABLES

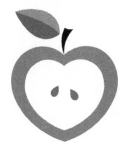

7 Steps to Healing After Loss

MARIE SCOTT

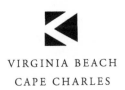

VIRGINIA BEACH
CAPE CHARLES

In Loving Memory of William David Scott.
Cheers to the life we shared and
the memories we made.

DISCLAIMER

THE INFORMATION SHARED IN this book is for educational and informational purposes only and is not intended to be viewed as medical or mental health advice. It is not designed to be a substitute for professional advice from your physician, therapist, attorney, accountant, or any other health care practitioner or licensed professional. The Publisher and the Author do not make any guarantees as to the effectiveness of any of the techniques, suggestions, tips, ideas, or strategies shared in this book as each situation differs. The Publisher and Author shall neither have liability nor responsibility with respect to any direct or indirect loss or damage caused or alleged by the information shared in this book related to your health, life, or business or any other aspect of your situation. It's your responsibility to do your own due diligence and use your own judgment when applying any techniques or situations mentioned in or through this book.

Table of Contents

FOREWORD

THERE ARE A FEW times in your life that you come across someone who makes you fall in love with life all over again. Someone who demonstrates deep gratitude and a zest for making the world a better place. Marie is just that person.

I met Marie many years ago as she was embarking on her journey to optimal health. Despite everything she had gone through personally, Marie always had a smile on her face and a radiant energy about her. It excites me to know that she will be sharing some of her lessons in this book.

Losing a loved one is never easy, and it can seem impossible to move forward without the right support system and community to guide you through the process. Often our health, relationships, and career struggle as a result of our loss. It can be very difficult to bounce back.

Marie has overcome her own personal adversity and turned it into a newfound passion to help others feel their best, mentally and physically. She took the powerful life lessons she learned from widowhood and functional medicine and has followed her passion to serve others by helping them find self-love, laughter, and the strength to move on.

She is one of the sweetest people you will meet and has a heart of gold. I'm so thrilled that she has captured her journey for others to reclaim their lives and love once again. In this book, you will find timeless principles of healing the body, mind, and soul. You will find new strength, discover new levels of health, and celebrate life once again!

SACHIN PATEL

PART 1

The End

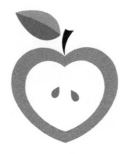

CHAPTER 1

Dave

It was a beautiful Sunday morning when the love of my life took his last breath in my arms. On April 15th, 2018, at 8:32 a.m., retired Captain William "Dave" Scott, of the Mississauga, Canada Fire Department, peacefully slipped away from this earth. He'd spent his last months trying to convince me that I would be alright without him—a sentiment I couldn't imagine after three decades together.

The moment he passed was simultaneously the most beautiful and most devastating moment of my life. I'd whispered in his ear that morning after the sleepless night before, "It's okay, honey, I'll be alright."

I lied.

The grief that comes after a loss to cancer is a bulldozer, shattering everything in its path. My entire life as I knew it was shattered into pieces. Never in my wildest dreams could I imagine life without him by my side; it never crossed my mind. After about twenty years of marriage, we used to joke, "Sweetie, want to grow old together?" and he'd say, "Too late!"

From the minute he passed, everything was different. Every. Single. Thing.

How many times have you heard the saying, "What doesn't kill you makes you stronger?" After Dave left this earth, I often laid down on the floor, staring at the ceiling. One day, I was in the sunroom on the floor with my arms open and empty, wondering, NOW who do I take care of? And the answer came back to me quickly—YOU silly!

After thirty years of being a dedicated Florence Nightingale to my beloved Dave, from his first knee scope in 1989 when they told Dave he'd never climb a ladder again (and he was determined to prove them wrong), through three brain surgeries, two knee replacements, two hip replacements, and finally the esophageal cancer that brought him down, I was a good nurse. I accompanied him to every single test, never left him alone in the hospital, drove him to rehab while he was on recovery drugs, took care of him, fed him well, picked up his meds, and tried to help him stay positive. After all the health challenges he'd overcome throughout his life, we thought he'd beat cancer with no problems.

Cancer is sneaky like that.

When my mom met Dave for the first time at the every-Sunday pasta dinner, she fell in love. Mom said, "Mangia Mangia" which means *eat* in Italian. And Dave did, as he had been a card-carrying member of the "clean plate club" since childhood. In an Italian household, as soon as you finish your plate, you get a heaping scoop of seconds. Boy was he stuffed that day as Mom and Dad kept piling pasta and meatballs on his plate. My brothers were just sitting there watching this happen and laughing to themselves. Is "death by meatballs" appropriate for a headstone? They welcomed him to the family with open arms and full bellies.

Family was important to Dave, and this led to the decision to make one last road trip up north from South Carolina where we lived for almost twenty years. He had some final goodbyes to say, not only to his family but to mine. We shared a lot of family losses in our time together. He lost his mom to cancer when she was only thirty-five. Soon after his dad retired at age sixty-two, he passed away. He lost his stepmom shortly after, sadly just as she was igniting a romance with a longtime friend. My brother was gone. My aunts and uncles are all gone, as were Dave's. Our immediate family became each other.

After Dave's diagnosis, we flew up to Rochester, rented a car, and the first stop was to see Mom. It brought both of us to tears which we tried to hide, but by then Mom's Alzheimer's was already so advanced that we didn't need to tell her why we were there. She did say to my sister the next day, "Dave's losing some weight."

Moms could always tell, couldn't they?

In all the years Dave and I were together, I'd call Mom and Dad every single Sunday, and without fail Mom would say, "Oh, hi Marie, how's Dave?" Without fail, and laughing, I'd say, "I'm fine, Mom, here's Dave." Mom never forgot her kids' names, or Dave's, but the grandkids and the great grandkids were a bit fuzzy as the years passed. My Dad died in April of 2010 and Mom passed in December 2018. We really lost Mom to her Alzheimer's when Dad died; she totally withdrew into herself.

Dave and I moved up to Rochester and stayed with her for six months after Dad passed. She couldn't be left alone by then, and we had to move her out of our childhood home we all grew up in at 88 Cherry Road and into a safe place where she had full-time care. The stress of aging parents can take a toll. Dave was right by my side the entire time.

The Saturday of our road trip my older sister Lin had everyone from my extended family over to her house. The event was a feast, of course, because total gluttony was how my family celebrated anything. I have four sisters: Marg, Kathy, Jean, and Lin. Dave commented many times over the years about how we celebrated every single occasion with food. That day my brother Rich said to me in private, "This is embarrassing, this feast," because by then Dave couldn't eat more than a bite of anything. I had three brothers: Rich, Mike, and my oldest brother George.

Dave had half a shrimp that day, and it didn't stay down. The days of "Mangia Mangia" were long gone. That night, we planned a little diversion to Seneca Niagara Casino where we were going to meet old friends Bob and Sue. He had a craving for french fries, so we stopped at a diner on the way to Buffalo, and he could barely get one down. It was a fun night at Seneca though.

Dave's last bite of his favorite meal was a tiny piece of ribeye that Bob ordered at the restaurant that night. At the club bar, I remember Sue running her hands through Dave's thick white hair and apologizing for doing it, but she didn't need to, because Dave loved it.

The next day, we drove up to Toronto and stayed at the Marriott Eaton Centre Hotel, and they upgraded me to a suite. From my decades of business travel, I earned status with lots of airlines and hotels. We had dinner with Dave's son Geoff that night in our suite and watched a Toronto Maple Leafs hockey game and just sat and talked. His son shared kind words and stories about him and thanked him for being a good coach to him as a kid. It got me thinking about how lucky we were to have the time to tell the people we love how we felt. Many people don't have that opportunity.

The following day, we saw his daughter Laura for the last time at Swiss Chalet for lunch. Swiss Chalet held special memories for us both. One of my first meals in Collingwood where we skied was at Swiss Chalet. I was a bit miffed when Dave DARED to take me to a CHAIN chicken restaurant! How dare he. I was hooked from that day on; every single trip to Canada, our first stop was Swiss Chalet. The only thing we ever ordered was a quarter white chicken with fries. At lunch with Laura, Dave could only have a couple of sips of soup. It was sad watching him at lunch, knowing he couldn't have his favorite "quarter white chicken" that day.

It was so hard and weird listening to him say goodbye to his children knowing he'd never see them again. The hugs were extra-long and emotionally draining.

The flight home from that trip north was very painful. Dave could hardly walk and had no energy. We couldn't find anything in any airport to drink or eat. I tried pleading with the TSA to let me through with an unopened bottle of Ensure, but the agent said, "Nope, can't do that, if we did, we'd have to let everybody through with something or other!" The agent was just doing his job, but the entire process was gut-wrenching.

So we settled for a single order of chicken fingers at a Buffalo airport restaurant. Dave could barely eat one.

Our final month together was spent with an outpouring of feelings of deep love. I only once said to Dave, like any good Italian wife, "You gotta eat!" As soon as it was out of my mouth, I regretted saying it.

I focused my attention in those last weeks on making him as comfortable as possible. I followed him around with little plastic cups, holding his head while he got sick quite often, because by then, he couldn't keep anything down, not even water.

I remember going into the bank to change our accounts over and sitting down in the banker's office. Dave had his cup and apologized in advance in case he got ill. The poor woman innocently said, "I hope it's not contagious." She almost bolted from her office. "Don't worry," we responded, "this isn't something you can catch."

Dave was in good spirits until the end, a remarkable feat for any mortal facing the end of their life. We lived every day in the moment, totally in the present, with little fear of the future.

Remarkably, Dave was more worried about me and how I'd live out the rest of my days. He confided in his closest friends about this worry, and we also talked about it on the front porch where we sat each night. It was hard for him to bring up the topic, but he was determined to make sure I gave myself permission to embrace life once I was ready, in whatever fashion I wanted.

Our dear friend Donna drove down to see Dave two weeks before he passed. This was her first road trip since her husband Marv died two years before. The four of us—Marv, Dave, Donna, and I—fixed up townhouses in Virginia and rented them out. We would stay at Marv's house for weeks on end while the renovations took place, and the four of us had wonderful dinners and many talks about everything under the sun. Marv was a beautiful soul, never afraid to speak his mind and offer his opinion with grace and humility.

Bill, Dave's old friend and favorite mechanic for over forty years, traveled down to see us on his way to Florida, for the first time, all the way from northern Ontario in Canada.

It was as if everyone knew Dave wasn't going to be in this world for much longer.

I asked our dear friend and nurse extraordinaire, Maryann, to give me a second opinion on ideas to help Dave. He started himself in hospice in March, thinking that it would give me help (me, not him!) when the time got near. We never dreamed for a minute that his time left was going to be so short.

We were four weeks away from the end.

Everything we tried up to that point wasn't easing Dave's constant heaving (mostly just saliva). I called Maryann one day and said, "You've given us one miracle back when he had his brain aneurysm years ago. Got another one in you?" Her husband Peter joined Maryann, and they arrived the Thursday before Dave died. Maryann met with our amazing and beautiful hospice nurse, Nicole, and they couldn't come up with any new ideas. Dave's color was so good, though, that Maryann started making plans to fly home to Phoenix the following Monday. Well, that didn't happen. Dave only made it to Sunday.

Dave never for one minute got angry about his diagnosis. Feeling sad—yes. I remember serving him his frozen Jell-O cubes made with a special nutrient rich protein powder (designed for gastric bypass patients), and I gave him four tiny cubes. He had tears in his eyes saying, "Honey, you know I can only eat three, but you gave me four." It breaks my heart to this day when I think about it. So, to parents out there, I protest, please banish the clean plate club forever.

The Saturday before Dave died was sunny and warm and we loved sitting on the back deck watching the golfers go by. People stopped by out of the blue, people called out of the blue, and it was like the universe put out a message to tell everyone, *check in with Dave*. Felix, a fellow firefighter from NYC, visited and sat on the back deck for an hour after golf. Cyndy came by with her dog Angel. Later,

Dave was crying that Angel was going to miss him, and she certainly does! Kathy and her dog Scout came by the front porch. Neighbor Carl brought over his famous grilled chicken, because he saw all the company I had, which was very thoughtful.

Dave's golfing buddy Dick, a retired pastor who he called "Rev," came and sat with him on the front porch; they called it "religion hour." The week before, Dave called the Rev and asked him to come over for an emergency religion hour. He told me later, Dave's biggest worry was about me and what I would do without him.

Dave was in his recliner late that afternoon and his right knee swelled up and turned black. Dave had allergic reactions to many things over our lifetime together, and we thought it was simply a reaction to something he was taking, maybe one of the meds in his compound cream. Because he couldn't swallow anything, not even a pill, his pain medications (morphine and other stuff) were compounded into a cream he could apply easily to his wrists. Maryann thought it might be a blood clot. He deteriorated quickly after that. Peter and Maryann helped me get Dave in bed that night, literally the three of us carrying and lifting him by his belt straps.

Later that night, I left the bed and went to the chair in the corner. He was so restless; I sat and watched over him from there. Since Maryann mentioned the blood clot earlier, we had propped his lower legs onto a pillow, and he was doing foot pumps in his sleep over and over.

At one point, he woke up as he often did and patted my side of the bed to make sure I was there. I wasn't. He said, "Honey, when I realized you weren't there, I had to feel my pulse to make sure I was still alive." This broke my heart and still brings me to tears to this day. I crawled back into bed and held him close the rest of the night.

About 6:00 a.m., I went and woke up Maryann for help; I somehow knew the end was near. We sat by him and held him close, lying in our bed. He was lucid almost right up to the end, just very, very weak. That last morning of his life as I held him for hours, he simply just stopped breathing, in my arms, at home like he wished.

8:32 Sunday morning, April 15, 2018.

Before he passed, I whispered in his ear "Dave, I'll be alright." I knew it was a lie, and I am sure Dave knew too.

On that Sunday morning, his last day on earth, Dave's best and oldest buds from Canada, Larry and Bob, were headed down to see Dave, but it was too late. They did end up turning around and headed back north after making it all the way to Pittsburgh. The next day our friends Bob and Georgette from Ontario were also headed down to see Dave. I had no way to get a hold of them, and they showed up at the door Monday morning. When they arrived, they were shocked at the news, but it was still good to see them, and I welcomed them into the house. They ended up staying a couple of days and made the best of the trip down and then back up to Canada.

That whole weekend was a blur and so painful. I remember being in shock, and I remember the constant stream of visitors that weekend. Of course, there was a ton of food brought into the house. We had such wonderful and generous friends and neighbors. All I could think about while receiving the food was how Mom, Dad, and brother George were together again with Dave up in heaven. I could hear Mom saying, "Mangia, mangia, Dave." Eat, eat!

Everyone told me for months after, "Oh you're so strong, you'll be fine." They didn't know what went on during the quiet nights or the quiet lonely mornings for at least the first year. That's the thing about grief, most people don't see you when it hits. They didn't see the lonely weekends, especially Sundays, all by myself in the house, not feeling so strong. Collapsing in the bedroom closet sobbing for hours on the floor, I'm not so strong. When I was on the road traveling for work, and I landed, and there's nobody to text that I've arrived, nobody to call right before sleep in my hotel room and say good night my love, I'm not so strong. When there was no one to come home to, no one to pick me up at the airport, and nobody to leave love notes for, I'm not so strong.

I never felt very strong at all. I felt tender and weak with a heavy broken heart.

CHAPTER 2

If You Wanted Easy, You Could Have Married Anybody

I can't tell you how often I heard the line *"if you wanted easy, you could have married anybody"* over the almost thirty years (twenty-nine and five months and five days, but who's counting?) Dave and I were married. I spent half my life with this larger-than-life man with no regrets.

I remember December 6, 1986, like it was yesterday, the day we met. Getting to Grey Rocks Ski Hill in Quebec from my hometown of Rochester, NY, should have been a direct bus trip with the rest of the Ski Huggers group, but not for me. It took planes, trains, a cab, and a bus.

Ski Huggers was a group (mostly singles) of downhill skiers who got together at the local ski hills in Rochester and for longer ski trips like Grey Rocks. I never got on the bus out of Rochester, because the night before I had too much fun celebrating my upcoming trip. So instead of meeting the group in the Xerox parking lot in Rochester, NY, on Saturday morning at 10 o'clock, I missed them completely by not waking up until 9:45 that morning. I was in a panic trying to figure out how I was going to get to Quebec. Had I sacrificed the ski slopes for too many drinks? I had prepaid for this fabulous all-inclusive ski trip six months earlier and had been looking forward to the trip so much that I was determined to get there.

The trip I almost didn't make was the trip that changed my life.

After waking up, shaking off the panic attack, and gulping down a coffee, I booked a one-way plane ticket out of Rochester, NY, to Montreal, Quebec. A train in Montreal took me to the bus station. I took a bus to the St. Jovite station next, and then a cab for the last leg to the Gray Rocks resort. Fortunately, back then I had no bulky ski equipment because I was going to rent everything, so I only had the clothes I needed for the week—ski suits, sweaters, and dancing clothes because a girl has always got to be ready to dance anywhere and anytime, even at the ski hill. When I finally opened the door to my room at Gray Rocks at two in the morning, my two roommates, whom I hadn't met yet, were not impressed! Was it the late entrance? Did I still smell like the party girl from the night before? I'll never know.

During the whole week at Gray Rocks, there were parties, events, and dancing every night in the bar. Early in the week I noticed this handsome, super friendly guy flirting and laughing and dancing with every woman there. I thought to myself, *he's trouble*, but I was intrigued anyway despite my initial impression.

On the last night of the trip, he asked me to dance. He made a comment that no one had been able to keep up with him on the dance floor all week, and I thought to myself *really? Perhaps you just picked the wrong dance partners all week?* The gauntlet was thrown down. I wore him out dancing, because I refused to stop. It was almost like a double dare, and I am known to be a little stubborn. I was pretty fit back then; it was my racquetball playing years. I knew my dancing shoes would come in handy. That was me, always prepared. I planned everything in my life, until the night I met HIM.

Dave asked for my number, and I gave him my work phone and no address other than somewhere in Rochester, NY. It was way before cell phones and before the internet was invented. I didn't have

Sir Google or social media to do background checks . . . but I had a gut feeling that this guy might be THE guy. Our meeting like this at Gray Rocks set the stage for many crazy and spontaneous adventures over the next thirty years.

I became a road warrior (before I met Dave) back when I entered the world of Human Resource and Payroll software with a company called Information Associates out of Rochester, NY. I was consulting with and teaching project teams who bought the software, designed for colleges and universities. I really think my early desire to be on the go and travel was due to "SAD" disease—Seasonal Affective Disorder. I realized when I was seventeen and took my first flight to NYC for my very first out of town date, that likely the only time I'd ever see the sun was in the air. USA Today had a daily little clip titled "Did you Know" which noted that Rochester, NY, had the dubious honor of being one of the ten cloudiest cities in the US! Little wonder I wanted to travel, and I did as often as I could. I still love traveling, whether it's for work, speaking, or pleasure. The best is a combination of all three!

During my time working with Information Associates in Rochester, I went back to night school and achieved my Associates Degree in Human Resource Management. I have a love of learning which Dave supported throughout our time together and which I still have. My alma mater was the Rochester Institute of Technology, and I graduated Summa Cum Laude. The only reason I did this in my twenties was to get out of a 9 to 5 payroll office job and start to travel as a consultant for the company. My manager at the time, Pete, believed in my dream and helped me to make it come true with Information Associates. After I graduated with honors, he promoted me, and I hit the road. Traveling became a pleasure, a dream, and a passion. I loved visiting new cities, big and small, and experiencing the different cultures (and food!) around the world. After I moved to Mississauga, Ontario, with Dave, and joined J.D. Edwards in 1990 as employee number nine in Canada, it kick-started my global travels. Later, throughout my thirty-year career with Oracle, I have been fortunate to travel across Canada, most states in the US, and globally to Italy, Copenhagen, Seoul, and South Korea (right before 9/11; I got home on 9/8). Eventually, Oracle bought this company, J.D. Edwards, and I spent nearly thirty years in my technology career.

In Rochester, I lived in a cute Cape Cod house on a street called Shady Way. It was my little touch of heaven. I was in my late twenties and having fun playing the field, not looking for anything long term, and neither was Dave. Finding love was not on my mind at all. About five months after the Quebec ski trip, Dave started calling me and asking me out to dinner. The first time he called he said, "You probably don't remember me," but I certainly did the second I heard his voice.

I made up an excuse that night for not going out. Part of me was excited and part of me was a bit reserved about jumping in with this man I had reservations about when I first met him five months before. I told him I had to do my laundry, and then he said, "I'll call tomorrow." And he did call, for the next four days, and the excuses ranged from I was too busy, I had to wash my hair, or I even used this one: my sister-in-law was having a baby (Andrew, my godson).

He was so persistent and persevering, I figured – well if he wants to take me out to dinner that bad, then let's do this. Not to mention, I ran out of excuses. It was May 2, 1987, our first date, and also the day Andrew was born. A while later, I found out Dave drove in from NYC where he had just broken up with his then-girlfriend (which is why it took so long to hear from him). He was a one-woman man and for some reason must have really liked those long-distance relationships, because we started another one that night.

Back then, there was no GPS and Dave didn't have my address yet because I didn't give it to him. He lived and worked in Mississauga, Ontario, right outside the city of Toronto. I told him to call me when he got close to my city of Rochester. Well, I couldn't believe this but when he called, he was exactly two blocks away from my house, at the cemetery buying flowers. Why the cemetery? There was always a flower vendor set up at each entrance of the cemetery, one entrance on Lake Avenue and one on Dewey Avenue, the main road I lived off, remarkably only two blocks away.

I gave Dave the address, along with verbal directions, and about two minutes later, I heard the Corvette (Dave's baby—1967 Stingray 357 metallic turquoise blue convertible) pull in the driveway about 4 PM. The doorbell rings and there's Dave, flowers in hand, wearing a sweaty white firehouse T-shirt. The first thing he said, after handing me the cemetery flowers and giving me a kiss on both cheeks, was "Hi! How are you? Mind if I take a shower?" How's that for an opening line?

For dinner, he was looking forward to a Caesar salad. Well, Rochester dining wasn't anywhere near the variety found in Toronto, so the search for a Caesar Salad was not as easy as you might think. Not to mention the iPhone with its ton of travel and restaurant apps, or the internet for that matter, hadn't yet been invented. Flowers from the cemetery, a shower, and a search for Caesar salad. There was nothing conventional about Dave from the beginning.

We ended up going to Agatina's for dinner, where I figured an Italian restaurant would be the best chance to find a Caesar, but they didn't have one. We had a fabulous and memorable dinner anyway. Instead of a Caesar Salad, we had the "Agatina's Italiano Salad" with romaine, chickpeas, Italian Ham, olives, salami, provolone, artichoke hearts, tomatoes, and Italian dressing. We shared a plate of what I later learned was Dave's favorite dish, Fettuccine Carbonara. Agatina's is still open, by the way, after all these years, plus they NOW have a Caesar Salad on their menu.

After dinner, we went to a club in downtown Rochester that was featuring a rock band of retired police and firemen. Fitting for a night out with a firefighter. This is also the first time Dave learned about how directionally challenged I was then and still am today. As I was navigating to the bar, we must have circled the inner loop highway about four times, and he finally said, "Didn't we just pass that same church again?"

I remember thinking after dinner and dancing that night, I can't let him drive three hours home to Mississauga, after his very long day, so I'll just let him sleep on the couch. True confession time—I've never told anyone this—we didn't leave the house for four whole days after that night. He left only because he was on duty and he had to get back to Mississauga for his night shift, while I just called in sick for those four days to my job at the time. I remember vividly to this day our first kiss in the dining room on Shady Way. He did sleep on the couch that night, and so did I. Love and lust at first sight.

Dave was born on January 21, an astrology sign of Aquarius, and he was nine years older than me. Capricorn and Aquarius were on the cusp the year he was born. If you know much about "horrorscopes" (Dave's term), then you might know an Aries (my sign) and Aquarius are together because of past lives, karma, and all that jazz. I am convinced there's some truth in that statement. Plus, he was the only guy who was not in the LEAST intimidated by my three protective Italian/Arab brothers all living in Rochester. And, he was the only guy I couldn't beat up. We wrestled all the time, and when I'd try to jump on him and tackle him to the ground, he'd laugh and say, "Is that a fly on my back?" One time at our house on Greenhurst in Mississauga, he threw me over his shoulder like I was a five-pound bag of rice, in an awesome fireman's carry, and started marching out the front door with me hysterically laughing and beating him on the back. The only problem was I had no clothes on!

The next date in Rochester was the week after his seven-day shift at the firehouse was over. We were walking on the pier in Charlotte Beach and the conversation turned out to be about what our ideal "job description" would be for a relationship. We both agreed love, trust, and laughing were the top three. We never wavered from these top three priorities for the thirty years we were together.

He also proposed to me on that second date walking the Charlotte Pier, even though every time I told the story over the years, he insisted he didn't propose—he TOLD me I was going to marry him. And he was right. We both knew our number was up, even though we both started this relationship with no desire for commitment, let alone to ever be married again. My only condition was that we get through all four seasons first, but I didn't last those four seasons like I thought I would. We only made it through three.

We shared planning special date weekends in the first year we were together. We never postponed adventures and never said let's wait until we retire, and I'm so grateful we lived life to the fullest. We had a "trip" jar, kind of like a bucket list, only a jar list. Both of us would put our suggestions in the big glass jar, and each month we'd pick one out. One early trip was Waterloo, NY, staying in an unusual "Cat Museum" in Geneva. The museum was attached to a delightful bed and breakfast, all marble throughout with paper slippers at the front door. I have the sweetest picture of Dave posing by the marble fireplace in the mansion suite. There was a patio out back where we were served a very intimate lobster dinner with fine wine. We were there visiting Mark Twain's hometown. Twain was one of Dave's favorite authors. Huckleberry Finn, the adventurer, had nothing on Dave. If Twain were still alive, they'd be drinking buddies for sure.

Another weekend trip was to the Corning Glass Factory where we watched how glass is blown from the experts. Dave bought me a beautiful Steuben glass vase which I still have on my office desk, etched with the saying, "Chance cannot change my love nor time impair." Our trip to Seneca Lake was a wine tasting tour, in a romantic log cabin right next to the wineries in the Finger Lakes region. Wine continues to be a passion of mine! We watched fireworks in Toronto on the lakeshore, set to classical music, every July. Toronto had the best celebrations, whether it was fireworks or the annual Canadian National Exhibition, we took advantage of everything we could in that wonderful gem of a city. If we weren't together doing something fun, we talked on the phone for hours every day and every night. We were determined to soak up every second of life even back then, and we were determined to do it together.

Dave proposed again, kind of, at the Sherwood Mall in Mississauga, four short months after we met. But we both knew it was meant to be by then, and even though I said we had to wait four seasons, I knew this was it and my single days were over. Dave and I were true soulmates, and both of us knew this relationship was different since that very first date.

We were walking around the mall, window shopping, and Dave innocently steered me into this jewelry store on our way to breakfast. Dave asked me if I saw anything I liked in the engagement ring section. I really didn't see anything that caught my eye, plus I wasn't expecting this to happen so quickly, and I said "No, nothing is calling out to me." He gave an imperceptible nod to the jeweler and he disappeared into the back room. He came out about five minutes later and handed a box to Dave. He opened it, and said, "how do you like this one?" Well, it was beautiful, and of course, it fit perfectly.

A while after Dave proposed on that second date, he said in his silly accent, "Darlin', quit your job, move in with me, and come skiing with me for the winter."

So I did!

So what if I had crushing student loan and credit card debt?

So what if I couldn't work in Canada?

So what if I really wasn't that good of a skier?

So what if I had to sell my lovely house on Shady Way?

Let's just start our life together with a great Dave and Marie adventure, he said, so I did. It turned out to be the best winter I ever had.

Peter and Maryann were our dearest best friends and a large part of our traveling adventures over the years. The Canadian Ski Patrol, and I'm sure the US Ski Patrol as well, is made up of a lot of firefighters and nurses. This is because they already have a lot of safety and first aid training knowledge and have a desire and love of helping people. They also have these crazy shifts that allowed them to ski in the first place during the week, with so many days off in a row. Maryann spent her career as a nurse, eventually becoming a traveling nurse after they moved to the US from Canada. Dave met them first, right after they got married. Peter and Maryann spent their entire winter there up in Collingwood (north of Toronto) celebrating their honeymoon. Dave always joked and told everyone he spent their honeymoon with them. Maryann and Peter were by my side when Dave had his brain aneurysm, by my side the last week of Dave's life on earth, and by my side when he took his last breath in my arms that Sunday morning. They were that close to us for all of our married life.

Many of the patrollers were also trained in emergency triage care, such as nurses like Maryann and firefighters like Dave. One day at Osler, we were skiing together, and as we were riding the chair up to the top, we spotted a lifeless body in the trees on a run near what was called the "old liftline." Dave flew off the chair and gave me instructions to yell to his fellow patrollers for help. A woman was badly injured, and as the first patroller in, he immediately began triage. He conducted a full exam and uncovered multiple injuries, including a skull fracture, damage to the eyes, hip, shoulder, and ribs, all later confirmed by the hospital. The injured woman did make a full recovery and praised the patrollers for their excellent treatment and kind words of reassurance. For this incident, Dave was so proud to be awarded the Douglas Firth Award, named after the founder of the Canadian Ski Patrol. That was Dave, always serving and helping others.

Our wedding was a spectacular event. It turned into a three-day celebration in Niagara Falls, NY. The reason why we picked the New York side over the Canadian side of the Falls was because the alcohol bill and the meal bill were WAY cheaper stateside. In fact, the party was not ready to stop at 11:00 p.m., and for a mere $100, we continued the open bar and music for one hundred thirsty guests (especially the Canadians). One of those Canadians from the ski patrol enjoyed the open bar so much that he passed out and was put onto a bar stool and carried all over the hotel. Pictures were taken. T-shirts were made afterwards.

My Mom baked fourteen beautiful trays of Italian cookies for the wedding, making sure there were enough left over for guests to take home in little brown baggies; that was the Italian thing to do. Mom was always in her element feeding people, and this was one more example of what made her smile and what she instilled in all of us with our love of cooking and eating.

Original wedding rings are irreplaceable. I still have my original ring, even after losing it for six months many years ago. I needed a mileage run to make Diamond frequent flyer status on Delta that year. The direct flight to New York City would put me over what I needed, and I talked my friend Cindy Chitty, who had never been to the "Big Apple," into joining me. We flew out on the 6:00 a.m. flight, landed at 7:30 a.m., and started our big one-day tour at the Empire State Building. It was December 30, the night before New Year's Eve, and the city was busy and buzzing, preparing for the big night. We took over two hundred pictures that day of all sorts of things we came across and did. This included spending the morning at the Empire State Building, being serenaded on the subway by a trio of Mexican Mariachi musicians, dinner in Little Italy, Wall Street, the famous Bull and Times Square (watching the ball being installed for New Year's Eve)—all in a single day. We went back to our hotel at the Hilton on Avenue of the Americas. I did make Diamond status on that trip, accomplishing my goal. Better yet, it was a great trip to be with such a good friend and to introduce her to one of our favorite cities.

It was only a one-night stay, so I only had one outfit. My routine every single night when I was on the road (I've been a road warrior for a very long time), was to take off the Rolex watch Dave bought me, along with my wedding ring, and set them side by side on the sink. We checked out of the hotel early the next morning and caught our early morning flight home. It was only after I got home that I realized my ring was missing, but oddly, I had my watch! I searched every single piece of clothing at least ten times, maybe one hundred times, looking in every single pocket, and scouring every inch of the bag I traveled with, but found nothing. We put a police report in after we called the Hilton and they couldn't find it either. We needed a police report in order to file an insurance claim. We did this months after the fact, because I was still searching everywhere, thinking it would show up. We filed the claim, insurance paid the claim, and Dave set the money aside in a separate account.

A couple of months after that, Dave and I were strolling in downtown Charleston during the famous annual Spoleto Festival, and a ring caught our eye in a local jewelry store. We both thought it was perfect, so we bought it! Well, about six months later, the closet rods collapsed in the master bedroom and everything had to be removed so Dave the handyman could reinforce the closet. When he was done, I was organizing and re-hanging all my clothes in the closet. It was after the last armful of clothes was going back into the closet that I just happened to look down, and I screamed. Dave came running and said, "What happened? Are you all right?" My wedding ring was lying there on the rug by the hamper. I have no clue where it might have been in that last armful of clothes and what pocket it might have fallen out of. How crazy is that? We immediately called the insurance company to give the claim back. You wouldn't believe how difficult it was to give the money BACK.

One work trip, I extended my stay to ski in Denver, where our company headquarters was back then. Dave was my fellow adventurer and flew into town because it was during his seven days off. His shift on the fire department was the "A" shift where he'd stay until he retired. Why was this important? As a firefighter, his shifts were predictable and set on a 28-day cycle. Every firefighter was on one of 4 shifts, A, B, C, or D Shift. The schedule for each shift was seven nights on, seven days off, four days on, four days off, four nights on, four nights off. That meant two weekends a month Dave was on duty as a Captain on "A Shift." That also meant he had seven whole days off in a row every single month. He traveled with me whenever he could. This was one of those times. We often joked that even though we were married for many years, it was really only a few years because of his shift work and my work travels.

Off we went to Copper Mountain. Copper was a very beautifully laid out ski hill with the runs set up by level of difficulty across the entire hill. After Gray Rocks, Dave took over being my teacher on the ski hill and he was a really good teacher. We got to this one run and he didn't realize it was a double diamond (the hardest level of ski trail) with moguls (mountains of snow built up). He would always ski down halfway and stop, look up, and wait for me to ski down to him. That was Dave, always checking in to make sure I knew my way. He told me afterward he looked up and said "Oh sh#%, either she's going to kill me or I'm going to kill her!" He yelled up the hill to me "do the hop-jump-turn" like he taught me. Hop-jump-turn, hop-jump-turn, hop-jump-turn and I did. It was one of the most memorable and exhilarating runs of my life. And when I got to him where he stood watching, I just kept on going, screaming at the top of my lungs whooping and hollering! What a thrill. We skied for years after that until I tore my knee up on the last run of the day on the last day of the ski year at Swain Ski Hill, outside of Rochester, which ended my skiing days and started our golfing days.

Dave was my best life coach. Since I was on the road a lot, virtually every single week of my entire career, my stress level was high. The stress came from traveling around the world, running projects, managing a team, and later carrying a sales quota as an account executive. When I was home, I loved to cook, and I'd be singing (badly) and dancing in the kitchen while creating and cooking up fabulous meals. He'd just laugh and leave me be, realizing it was good for my soul and good for my stress level. Plus, he loved my cooking! Dave was also the best career coach a girl could ever ask for. He was my support, had my back, knew my goals, and pushed me to better myself throughout my career.

One of the most memorable promotions was in a role as client manager. I got to build an incredible team of consultants who are all successful to this day. I'll never forget Dave's advice, telling me, "Being a manager/leader is not rocket science." I will never forget my team giving me a tiny little six pack of hot sauce with a card I still carry around calling me the "best and hottest manager ever." That year I took part in the "Leadership Challenge" course and was rated as one of the top leaders in Canada. Dave was so proud of me, becoming a manager and a leader just like him. It wasn't rocket science after all. Just treat people really well, point them in the right direction, give them the right tools, and get the heck out of their way.

We never went to bed mad, because Dave wouldn't let it happen. In our early days, my passion used to rage hot (usually once a month). I'd stomp and storm and leave the house in a huff, and Dave would say, "You can't just keep running away from me." And he was right. We settled down after those first few years and never went to bed angry. Dave used to tell me, "I love the passion in you, and I know it goes both ways, and that's why you can never have a gun."

He could imagine me making a great dish, which took a lot of time (like my awesome lasagna), and if our guests were eating and not enjoying it, he'd envision me saying, "What do you mean you don't like my lasagna?" Then the gun would come out, and I'd be put in jail for attempted murder.

The two of us did have some knock-down-drag-out fights, but they quickly melted away, and we could never remember what worked us up into such a frenzy to begin with. If we could remember, they were trivial like moving dirty coffee mugs around after I put them in the dishwasher or leaving the cap off the toothpaste. In my opinion, I think that's a sign of a good strong marriage, boiling over with emotion but then always making up. Dave could be a tough guy, and I understood that about him. With all the pain and suffering he experienced on the job, it was understandable. And I could be a tough gal too—hot headed Italian mixed with half Lebanese blood. This should be taught in high school: never go to bed angry! With anyone, yourself, your spouse, your friends or family. Also make sure the guns are locked up if I bring dinner (especially my favorite dish to cook, lasagna) over to your house and you don't like it!

"Home is where your honey's suitcase is" was our favorite saying. We loved to travel, and loved to experience new things, dine on new foods, meet new people, visit new places, and make new memories. It was this way from the very first time we met in Quebec on that epic ski trip, right through to Dave's last months. I even surprised him and made his final bucket list happen, a flying lesson. We also enjoyed our quiet times every night and every morning together, reading the paper or just sitting on the front porch watching the world go by.

One beautiful morning in Sydney, Australia, we went to Bondi Beach. Back then I wore glasses at least an inch thick to read. I was sitting on the beach reading for what seemed like hours, and when I sat up, I noticed Dave with this cute smile on his face. I looked around and noticed no one had clothes on except us, and I smacked him on the arm with my book and said, "What were you thinking!" Both of us left shortly after, laughing, with our bathing suits still on. This scene repeated itself when we were on an all-inclusive beach vacation in Jamaica. We got in late the evening before and the next morning, when we flung open the curtains, eager to have coffee on the balcony, lo and behold, there we were again, overlooking a nude beach. We gingerly closed the curtains, hoping no one would notice we were dressed, went back into the room, and didn't venture out there again the rest of the week.

I came home one day in 1998 from work and announced I needed a change! It was time to move stateside for a lot of different reasons. The biggest reason being I was hitting the top of the foreign tax credit allowance which meant I was getting close to paying taxes in BOTH countries which was not cool. Dave was fast approaching his thirty years with the fire department which meant he could retire with a full pension at age fifty, plus he said he didn't feel "lucky" on the job anymore. It was a horrific year for him, from a baby's death, a rolling garage floor collapse, and multiple fires. I could see the stress of these traumas mounting on him and his beloved crew of men.

One of the things I am most grateful for is that Dave enjoyed the heck out of over twenty years of retirement because of our move to the United States. He didn't have to work, golfed four or five times a week, and traveled with me all over the place. His golfing buddies who were still working joked and asked how they could get a gig like that! We'd pack up the truck and just hit the road on a whim. No kids, no pets, fake plants (my favorite saying), allowing us to be without ties and able to lock up the house and go. When asked how he was enjoying retirement, he'd respond by saying he didn't know how he ever found time to work.

We took monumental road trips that just seemed to happen every summer or fall, usually with no more than a week's notice. Our longest road trip we logged 3,085 miles, up to Canada and back. I tracked and marked each leg of the trip on Google maps, printed it to share with friends and family. We told the stories from that trip for years. We made sure one stop was always in Rochester to see Mom (we never missed seeing Mom on any trip up north) and then we meandered our way back home. We drove about six or seven hours a day, finding a great town to spend each night in and having a fine dinner in the best restaurant we could find. No fast food for us!

Recently, a Facebook memory popped up of another epic mileage run. A mileage run is a "trip to nowhere" to gain frequent flier miles. It was getting close to the end of the year and I had only made Platinum status on Delta Airlines, similar to my flight to NYC. I was spoiled the year before by reaching Diamond status, the highest frequent flyer level.

I found this incredible flight deal which took me halfway around the world on a frequent flyer forum, talked it over with Dave, and he said, "Go for it!" He knew it was THAT important. We both benefited from my diamond status the year before, since 95% of the flights I took or we took together, one or both of us would get upgraded. I loved giving Dave my first-class seat so he could be more comfortable with his broad shoulders.

Off I went on my mileage adventure. It was a Friday in December, and of course Dave drove me to the airport like he always did. I flew to Atlanta which is a major Delta hub. (My neighbor Eason said even when he dies, he's going to have to transfer through Atlanta.) From Atlanta it was off to Johannesburg, South Africa, where I was upgraded to a lovely Delta One flatbed seat for a fifteen-hour flight. I was fed very well, had a few glasses of wine (I love the word "few" as it can mean any number after a "couple"), watched about four movies, plus I had a Netflix series downloaded on my iPad. I only got about one hour of sleep, and landed in the most beautifully decorated (for Christmas) airport where I spent the next five hours. I am also a member of Delta's Airline Clubs which has always come in handy for any layover of forty-five minutes or more. They had a wonderful selection of African dishes on the buffet, salads, meat dishes, soups, and showers! My next stop in Amsterdam airport was also full of shops with Christmas decorations everywhere, but I headed right to the Delta SkyClub. I took a shower in a beautifully appointed marble shower room, and then had a wonderful meal there. I think my layover there was only three hours and then I was off home to Atlanta where, of course, I took a shower in the Delta SkyClub and flew home on Sunday night. All in all, it totaled 22,500 miles, three days in the air, five flights, four different airports, and I reached my goal of Diamond status.

I have a large world map that has been with me since my travels began. The map has colored dots on all the places I have been around the world. The rules were, you had to sleep over, spend the night, or have sex in that city. My mileage run didn't count toward a dot on my world map though, because a sleep-over or sex never happened. I should have changed the rules, since it was my map, to include cities you took a shower in. Then there would be two more dots on the map.

Sometimes you feel you're in control of life and plans, until you're not. You never think you're going to be alone. Dave often used to believe in the phrase *"Life is what happens while you're busy making plans,"* and he repeated it often. All of a sudden, all of those plans are upended when you become one, never to be the same again.

Sweetie, want to hear the song of the day? Music was one of Dave's greatest loves of his life. Besides me, of course. But seriously, Dave knew every word to every song written since 1960. On the other hand, I knew the first line of thousands of songs. And I'd make the rest up. I'd wake up every morning with a song in my head and I would turn excitedly to Dave and say, "Sweetie, do you want to hear the song of the day?!" And he'd put his fingers in his ears and groan with a smile on his face, "Noooooooo," but I sang it anyway. Before he knew it, he was humming my butchered song of the day, and then singing it, with all the right words of course. One of the songs that I woke up with quite often for some reason was "Moon River." I would start singing in the shower *"Moon river, wider than the sky"* and it would just bug the heck out of him because that's all the words I knew. I often joked with him that I should've been like Charlie Sheen on *Two and a Half Men* and become a ditty writer. Ditties are short and only two or three silly lines, just like my made-up songs.

Music was a HUGE part of our life.

I particularly like pretending I could sing opera in the shower. One day when we lived on Dixon Woods in upstate NY, I was singing loudly (and badly) in the shower, with the windows open, at the top of my lungs. Dave was working in the front yard of our two acres of heaven, and he heard the neighbor screaming to the kids, "STOP YOUR SCREECHING." Little did she know it was me in the shower and not her kids! Dave knew it was me, turned his head, and just laughed and laughed. He told that story many times.

Dave LOVED to play the spoons and sing at the top of his lungs. This actually started way back when I had a project in St. Johns, Newfoundland. I spent about six months there as an Oracle Sales

Rep for an account which I ended up winning (they are still a happy customer). There is a street in St. Johns called George Street, a party street, lined with bars and restaurants. Every pub and bar had entertainment every single night of the week. From the city website, they describe George Street as having the most pubs and bars per square foot than any other street in North America. I love this line from the city's website: *"This is George Street, where morality and your liver come to die."* We ended up at an Irish bar one night and Dave found himself a set of spoons and the love affair began.

One year on St. Patty's day at our clubhouse, there was a local two-person band entertaining us before and after dinner. Well, Dave asked the kitchen to get him two spoons and he sat there and played for hours. The band actually thanked him because people came up and started leaving tips for them for the first time that night.

Movies were a big part of our life as well. For us, going to the theatre meant sharing a big tub of buttered popcorn which we usually polished off before the movie started. The first movie we saw in 3D was "Avatar" and we became fans of those funny glasses you had to wear. We watched a lot of movies, more so than regular television shows. Dave discovered this one movie quite by accident one night on HBO called *Searching for Sugar Man*. It was an incredible story about Sixto Rodriguez who was born in Detroit and faded into obscurity after recording two music albums. The albums bombed in the US but found unbelievable success and a huge audience in Apartheid-era South Africa. Two people were determined to find out his fate and set about searching for Rodriguez. They found him still living in Detroit working in construction, and proceeded to write an Oscar award-winning documentary. Dave made all our friends watch Sugarman, (along with the music video *"Bring Me Sunshine"*). We must have watched the movie at least seven or eight times, never failing to have tears in our eyes at the end. It's a beautiful story, and the music is awesome. We golfed often with Dennis and Marilyn, and when Dave would make an amazing putt, Dennis would call him

Sugarman. It made Dave happy to see other people share his love of this movie. Dave felt Sugarman's influence on the issues in South Africa to be amazing. The story of the search, and then finding him, was very moving.

Tombstone was another favorite movie. Val Kilmer was one of our favorite actors, and he had a famous line, "You're my daisy!" We watched that movie at least ten times and Dave would turn to me and say, "You're *my* daisy!" A couple of months after Dave died, I opened the front door in the morning one day to say hello to the world, and what did I find on the front porch? A little yellow silk daisy. It took my breath away, and my heart skipped a beat. My friend Brooke calls these moments "God Winks" from Dave. Be open-minded and aware when these God Winks come to you when least expected, and hopefully they'll make you smile like they do me.

The very first Performance Club trip I won for work in the early '90s was to Kauai. We had a list of adventures to sign up for, and I thought a golf tournament would be a fun event, so I signed up for the two of us. I had never swung a club in my life, but Dave had been golfing since he was a teen, up until he got so mad at his game that he threw his clubs in the pond one day. I hired the golf pro that morning, saying to him, "You have to teach me every single thing I have to know to get me through a round of golf." He taught me everything from the grip, the stance, and the swing to important etiquette tips. This was the start of our love of golf together—every single weekend for us as a couple and three or four times during the week for Dave with the guys after he retired. We traded in our snow skis for golf. Added bonus: you need to wear way less clothes for golf than skiing.

The constellations have always fascinated me, and I've studied them since I was a teenager. I got Dave interested in them too. Okay, maybe for just a few of them, like the Big Dipper and Orion The Hunter. Orion became our favorite, partly due to the funny movie, *Beetlejuice,* and partly because Orion seemed to fill the sky, just like Dave's larger-than-life presence. It is spelled differently, but

Betelguese is the brightest star in Orion's belt. Whenever I traveled and when we talked together at night, we'd both look up at the sky and compare star notes. We both saw Orion together many times. It was very special when we did, and even today when I look up and see "the Hunter," it makes me smile.

This book began as a journal; it was therapeutic to jot down all the memories of our life together. I loved to write at the beach—my special place. One night when I was alone writing at Folly Beach in South Carolina (called the "Edge of America"), I sat on the balcony outside looking up at—you guessed it—Orion, filling the sky. It was a very clear night, and all of a sudden, one little tiny cloud went floating by Orion. One single cloud, and I knew it was a wave from Dave.

We LOVED cruising, it had all our favorite likes and vices in one place. Oceans, entertainment, dancing, whale watching, drinking, gambling, food, and no driving! We've cruised many places, and our memorable trips included Rome, Venice, Berlin, St. Petersburg, Copenhagen, Stockholm and the Amalfi Coast. Back in our early years, Dave always said he'd never go anywhere they didn't speak English. His mind changed with our first trip to Copenhagen where I had a work engagement and he joined me. The work part was three days, and I extended our stay to eight. If you had a job like mine and didn't take advantage of extending these trips to enjoy new places, tying work with pleasure and new adventures, then why travel? Travel is for sharing and making memories together and we created a lot of memories which I still hold dear.

Some of those memories came flooding back to me while I held him tight and close as he took his last breaths that Sunday morning. Memories of restaurant matchbooks he'd written love notes on to memories of his little black book with "nice legs" written by my name. Thousands and thousands of pictures, to all the ups and downs and love and loss we shared during our time together. Memories to be cherished forever. So much love, Dave, and so grateful to have experienced such unconditional love.

I still have the matchbooks with the love notes.

Was our time together perfect? Hell no! Was it funny? Hell yes! He always made me laugh and smile, even up to the last morning of his life April 15, 2018, when I was searching and texting the neighborhood for a wheelchair because he just wanted to get out on the front porch one last time.

The thought in my mind was, he was right, if I wanted easy, I could have married anyone.

CHAPTER 3

The Final Battle

"Sir, you'll have to step aside for a full body pat down."

How many people do you know who have had four brain surgeries, two knee replacements, and two hip replacements? When we traveled and went through airport security, Dave lit up the security machines like a Christmas tree. He always wanted to ask for the cute female agent for his full body pat down, but thankfully never said it out loud. I would have been bailing him out of jail for sure.

I was a good Florence Nightingale. The first time I went to the doctor in the early years with Dave was for his knee arthroscopy. The doctor told him he'd never climb a ladder again and therefore never work again, and he discovered his willpower and the power of rehabilitation, before and after surgery. Dave was an emotional man, and when he came out of the hospital that day in a wheelchair, he was in tears and swore he'd not stop working, because he wasn't ready to stop working, dammit! Through really hard work and lots of rehab, he did get back to the Firehouse for ten more years until he retired on his own terms. Someone else might have said, oh good, I can have an early retirement, but that wasn't Dave. Since that day of his first knee scope, I did things I never thought possible as his nurse and caregiver. This coming from the wuss (me) who couldn't stand the sight of blood or pain, mine or anyone else's.

Dave ended up in the hospital a LOT! If anyone would have an allergic reaction to anything, it was going to be him. His lips would swell, his face would puff up, and I knew that was my cue to get him to the Emergency Room. One time in Rochester his blood pressure dipped precariously low while he was taking a new medication. I tried getting him to lie down in bed so I could figure out what to do. It fell so low when he got himself up into the bathroom without me, he proceeded to faint. I ran to the bathroom from the closet and managed to hold his head from slamming into the back of the cement hard porcelain toilet and eased him to the ground. Emergency Room here we come again. When I arrived at the front desk, they asked me what was wrong, and before I could get a word out, he fainted, as if on cue. They rushed him right back to a bed in the ICU. He was admitted for the next seven days that time, with edema swelling over his whole body. You could actually watch the hives pop up everywhere and float over his skin. Once he healed, they had to teach him how to eat again because his throat was constricted from the swelling.

The doctors finally diagnosed him with "vasovagal" syndrome. I find it interesting this happened ten years before his burst aneurysm. It made me wonder if the two events were somehow connected. The only lasting symptom from this event was if he took a sip of his scotch on an empty stomach, he'd sneeze! Leave it up to Dave to have that kind of symptom.

Dave's first of four brain surgeries happened when he was twelve years old. He got slammed in the head with a golf club which resulted in a lot of reconstruction and a plate in his head. The next brain event which almost took his life, was on Election Day in November, 2008. I was in Myrtle Beach to attend the annual Payroll Conference for my fourth year straight, and Dave always came with me since it was a short three-hour drive north. Peter and Maryann, our oldest friends as a couple, lived on a golf course in Myrtle Beach. We were staying at our timeshare on the beach and planned to golf and have dinner with them afterwards at their home course, Myrtle Beach National. We always went a couple of days early to enjoy their company, and that Tuesday we had an early morning tee time. When we got to the number six tee (coincidentally this was their "home hole" where they lived and was the same as our home hole on our golf course in Summerville, South Carolina, hole number six), Dave teed up his ball, screamed, held his forehead, and dropped to the ground facedown like he was having a seizure. Nurse Maryann rushed into triage, rolled him on his side, kneeing him in his back to keep him breathing while I ran to the golf cart to dial 911. Ever try to dial a cell phone with a golf glove on, a shaking hand, adrenaline rushing through your system and panic in your heart? Well, you can't. At that exact moment, Maryann's neighbor looked out the window, noticed Maryann on the ground, and rushed out the door. Maryann screamed to her, "Call 911!!" The fire department arrived within two minutes, and stabilized Dave on the ground. Dave came to, and wanted to get up and keep golfing. The firefighters said, "Dave, calm down, we think you've had a stroke, let us take care of you like you'd take care of any one of us." Magic words from one firefighter to another, it calmed him right down and he let them care of him.

Dave described it as if he'd been hit on the back of his head with a baseball bat. That started the journey with two different hospitals in Myrtle Beach and both saying to us, "We can't help him, get him to Charleston." Both of us were in disbelief as to what was happening. Dave seemed fine, was lucid and talking normal, and only had a bad headache. Looking back, I remember Dave having bad headaches our whole life together, never thinking to have his arteries checked in his head. Who would ever think to do that anyway?

An ambulance transported him the two hours from Myrtle Beach to Charleston. The EMT's said, "Do you mind if we turn on the lights and sirens?" To which Dave replied, "Sure, if you don't mind me getting sick all over your ambulance!" Dave won that one. He still had his sense of humor even though he was in pain.

The first night in Charleston at MUSC (Medical University of South Carolina), the on-call doctors told me he wasn't going to make it through the night and suggested we make final goodbye calls. I still can feel the disbelief, pain, shock, and agony as Dave and I made those calls. With his voice breaking, and me shaking like a leaf, we made calls to his son and daughter in Canada, explaining he had a "brain bleed" and the doctors didn't think he'd make it through the night. I couldn't begin to fathom what those calls must have felt like to him; we never talked about it again.

How could all of this have happened so quickly? From having a headache, wanting to finish his golf game, to possibly not making it through the night—it was all panic inducing. They kicked me out shortly after, because visiting hours were over, and they began prepping Dave for emergency brain surgery. As I was leaving the hospital in a daze, numb as a zombie, shaking like a leaf, the anesthetist came chasing after me. He was asking me frantically if Dave was on any illegal (or legal) drugs at all because they were doing an emergency craniotomy in the morning. This further induced a sense of panic and dread. Dr. Ellegala, the brain surgeon who ended up saving Dave's life, intervened about 11:00 that night. He called me at the hotel I was staying at near the hospital, calmed me down, and called off the panic attack. He told me to meet him at 6 o'clock in the morning. He drew me a picture on a piece of paper that I still have in a Dave "brain" file. He said, "50% of people who have brain aneurysms that occur where Dave's was, in the Circle of Willis (the command center at the base of the brain), never make it to the hospital, 25% of the ones that do make it to the hospital don't make it out, and the remaining 25% survive but almost always with lasting neurological damage." He basically said there was little chance Dave would pull out of the surgery with no damage, or even alive. There was also a strong chance of another stroke induced by the surgery.

My heart stopped when I heard this. The doctor was so kind and compassionate though, he put me at ease and gave me trust that he was the best to handle this situation. We agreed the "clipping" of the aneurysm with a titanium clip was the best option. My friends, by my side through the whole ordeal, gathered around me in the waiting room and took me out to lunch at a restaurant close to the hospital. It was good to take my mind out of the waiting room for a while.

About seven hours later, Dr. Ellegala came out of surgery, still in his scrubs, with a HUGE smile on his face and told us the surgery was a success. He put a titanium clip on the burst aneurysm and then moved on to getting the blood out of the brain. Dave would be in Intensive Care for two more weeks, as the doctors put him on the "Triple H" therapy. This stood for hypertension, hypervolemia, and hemodilution. This therapy is used for patients with aneurysms secured by surgical clipping (like Dave's) to reduce the risk of rebleeding. One detail about Dr. Ellegala I'll never forget is how long and thin his fingers were—just what you want in your brain surgeon.

Dave was in the very secure and locked down wing of the Intensive Care Unit of MUSC, and since they would only allow me two hours a day visitation, I had a lot of time on my hands. That year I also went back to college (SUNY Empire State, remotely) to complete my bachelor's degree which I started way back in the '80s but never finished. It was always a personal goal on my bucket list and of course Dave was my biggest supporter. Courses began while Dave was in the ICU, and Spanish was my first course. That was pretty easy to handle with my limited brain capacity at that very stressful time. I did finally graduate with honors (just like my Associate's Degree, Summa Cum Laude) after two years of night school. We did go up to Saratoga Springs for the graduation. I remember my friend Terry asking me if I was going and when I said yes, I wouldn't miss it for the world, she said to me laughing, "You're going to be the highest paid graduate in that line!"

It was a miraculous recovery, according to the entire team of doctors. I wasn't convinced it was that miraculous though. During those two weeks in the hospital, he was hallucinating, talking wildly about crazy things, and in and out of consciousness. I was scared he wasn't going to pull out of this one at all. Every day I would head to the hospital and they would unlock the unit and let me enter. I stayed at either a nearby hotel or one of my friends would drive me to the hospital for the night visit (my eyesight is terrible at night). I spent the short two hours by his side, all I was allowed to visit. I was so upset they wouldn't let me be with him every minute of every day and night.

When Dave was finally released from the intensive care unit, the first stop on the way home was to his favorite barber Rick. The craniotomy where they cut Dave's head open from his left ear to the top of his head required shaving his beautiful mane of thick white hair. But they only shaved one side. He looked like Michael Keaton in *Beetlejuice*, wild and crazy. Rick fixed him up with a short haircut all around. Over the next six months, his hair almost all fell out due to the radiation from the frequent MRIs to check his head arteries. It did eventually grow back, thicker than ever.

Dave, for the rest of his life, swore they put his head on crooked. He'd take his glasses off and put them on the table and the glasses were always uneven and he'd say, "See, they're crooked!" I used to joke with him that at least he hadn't sprung a leak where they stitched his head back together.

My foray into social media started that year. I discovered a blog tool that let me have a global reach to everyone across the US and Canada thinking and wondering about Dave's health status. So many people signed on and kept track. I couldn't believe the reach of social media at that time. The blog still exists, proving that anything you post online lasts forever. It also rekindled my love of journaling which I find very therapeutic. In fact, this book started as a journal.

The first work trip I had after Dave returned home and was somewhat recuperated was to San Antonio, Texas. I hadn't traveled in a couple of months, the date was December 16, and I was very nervous and on high alert about leaving him alone. Dave was my life, love, and top priority. If he so much as held his breath too long, so did I. That morning I woke up early and was in the downstairs office working on my presentation. I was in sales, and my role was to deliver demonstrations of our Human Resource software to large companies. Dave was upstairs, and I heard a big BOOM. I swear I thought he fell on the floor and my heart started racing, and then I thought maybe a truck hit the house. I ran upstairs to check on him and he was okay. It ended up being a mild earthquake that hit our town of Summerville, South Carolina, that day, and we learned we lived on a fault line so it was due to happen again and again. Mystery solved.

I headed to San Antonio for the presentations, and we did end up winning that customer over to our software. This led to a trip to Copenhagen to "meet the parents" of this new customer, and Dave wanted to join me. This trip was nerve-racking since it was only three months after he came home from his burst aneurysm, and I wasn't sure he had totally recovered. I had my eyes on him the whole trip even though it was only six hours across the pond. I was so worried his head would explode, adding to my stress and anxiety in my role as chief caregiver. The ongoing concerns were the remaining aneurysms which hadn't been treated yet. Plus, his blood pressure was all over the place when he was released, and at first they had him on these high dose salt pills which caused it to spike one time to 200/100! Way too high, so off we went to the emergency room again the next day. They finally decided to take him off the salt pills; it was part of the "Triple H" therapy for brain aneurysms. I often wonder if they're still using this protocol.

I had nothing to worry about though. My fellow adventurer Dave had a blast with his free days touring all over Copenhagen. I was working with longtime friends and co-workers Kevin and Matt, and Dave became the team's tour guide on that trip. He'd go out walking and exploring the city every day and found cool spots and restaurants for us to return to after our work day was over. The guys asked Dave to buy them T-shirts at the Carlsberg brewery on one of his outings. I still have mine in the original bag in the closet, but it's an XL which was my size at the time. Maybe I'll get it out and wear it as a sleep shirt.

When the burst aneurysm was clipped, they knew there were three more which didn't burst yet but had to be fixed. One was calcified so they left that alone. For the other two, we scheduled an angiogram to have those "coiled" where they would fill the artery with thin wire, similar to a stent. Dr. Turk took over from Dr. Ellegala for the follow-up and he did the coiling shortly after we returned from Copenhagen. I was in the waiting room that morning with friend Cindy Chitty by my side, and the doctor came out with a printed X-ray of Dave's brain, with four different views. Dr. Turk, beaming with pride, starts excitedly telling me about the success of the coiling and the procedure he used, and finally I had to say, "That's great, but how's Dave?" Dave came through it with flying colors, of course. His golf game improved tremendously after that and the first time he broke eighty the guys said, "We want the same surgery you just had!"

He was monitored regularly with an MRI every six months. The doctor reminded us each time of how rare his full recovery was. Some of the common neurological symptoms after a burst aneurysm included speech issues, thinking problems, partial paralysis, muscle weakness, or numbness. The only issue Dave had was while eating; about 90% of the time, his knife would be upside down. He'd slyly look up at me out of the corner of his eye to see if I caught it, and we would both laugh. Dr. Ellegala, the brain surgeon, would laugh as well, and said if that's the worst symptom you have, that makes you a very lucky man!

I joined the brand-new YMCA near our house when it first opened up a couple of months after Dave recovered from his brain aneurysm. I never went at first, but he did. He would do one thing and one thing only—ride the bike. Three times a week, always while reading a book he had gotten from the library. Once a year when the Tour de France was on, he'd watch it at the gym and pretend he was riding along with them. Dave never missed one day of the Tour. Since he discovered it, he watched every single minute either live early in the morning, or the replay in the afternoon. It was a stunning beautiful scenic ride around countries most of which we hadn't visited yet.

The first of four surgeries for two hips and two knee replacements started while on one of our Canadian adventures and we ended up golfing in Ontario. All of a sudden, Dave couldn't finish the round, his hip hurt so bad. It crushed him not to finish eighteen holes. That was the beginning of many surgeries. Dave started working hard at the YMCA before each surgery with lots of "pre-rehab" working out at the gym, on the bike, trying to strengthen the surrounding areas. Dave had plenty of cortisone shots too, thinking they would help him avoid surgery, but that's not how it was going to work out. After the first full knee replacement, he was up and about in six weeks flat and back golfing with the guys. The hip was next, then the other knee and finally the last hip.

For that last hip replacement, Hurricane Mathew decided to rear his ugly head and bore down on our home near Charleston, South Carolina. We decided to evacuate because Dave didn't need to be at home where he'd be tempted to do more than he should, especially if power was lost and with him still on pain medications. We evacuated to Atlanta, about a six-hour drive away, and had a really fun weekend. In Atlanta we took a golf cart tour of the city, and ran into a gay pride parade. On one side of the street the Bible waving crowd stood, with lots of rainbows and diversity on the other side. Fortunately, it was very peaceful, not to mention colorful. Driving home we saw tons of trees littered along the road to home, and throughout our golf course neighborhood. Power did go out for a whole day so it was good we left.

Dave was put on a different blood thinner for the last knee replacement. It was called Eliquis, and as usual we read the entire contraindication sheet listing the side effects, and one thing stuck out. It said, if you shave and cut yourself, then you will die. Okay, it might not have been that dramatic, but that's how we took it. No one wants to survive everything he did only to be taken out by a papercut or a shaving nick. So, Dave grew a beard. He always had a mustache in his early years in the fire department, but he shaved it off in our third year together. Well, the beard was awesome, I loved it, and he kept it even after he stopped the drug.

"Honey – Deb wants to sell her house!"

For many years I always told Dave we needed to move into a house with the master bedroom on the first floor while we could, not wait until we HAD to move. My friend Deb and I were working out with our trainer at the YMCA, on June 4, 2017. Dates are meaningful in this chapter, because time accelerated quickly from this date forward. On our way to the gym, Deb made some mention of moving closer to her son, and I reminded her that we always told her we would buy her house in a "New York second." She said, "But you don't know what I'm going to ask for it." I said well, I do have an idea, and the number I had in my mind matched *exactly* the number that she had in her mind. Before we went in for our workout, I texted Dave and said *you won't believe this, but Deb is selling her house, and this is what she's asking.* (Please forgive me Dave, but I told you it was $10,000 more than what she wanted because I knew you'd insist on negotiating.) The next morning at the breakfast table, we let Dave negotiate the price down to what Deb and I knew it was going to be in the first place. We shook hands and had a deal. In one single day, a decision was made. Let me just say that Dave was not a quick decision maker and totally resisted change. I first learned this in Canada when we lived in the town of Mississauga in a one-bedroom house. It took three years before he agreed to move into a bigger place and to finally get my furniture from my house in Rochester out of storage. The fact that he made this decision so quickly to buy Deb's house makes me wonder to this day if he knew something was wrong. Once he passed the age of his dad, he thought he was in the clear to live for a long time after. His Mom died at age thirty-five from cancer, and his Dad also died from cancer at a young age shortly after he retired from the railroad in Canada.

I believe in my heart Dave knew then what we were up against.

This move was literally around the corner from our old house. Everybody thought the move was because of Dave and his health and medical issues, but it really was because of me. Our master bedroom was upstairs, and each trip, whether it was business or pleasure, I'd be hauling our luggage up and down the stairs for both of us. I was so scared of the stairs after my fall when I tore my rotator cuff that I really wanted to find a house with a master bedroom downstairs. And I wasn't so healthy myself back then.

We had lived on Peninsula Pointe in Summerville, South Carolina, for fifteen years, which was the longest we'd ever lived anywhere. You tend to accumulate a lot of stuff in fifteen years. I alone had four closets worth of clothes in all the sizes that I had been since Dave and I met. I went from a size eight back in the '90s and blossomed to a size twelve back in 1998 where I remained for the next twenty years. I felt that if I threw away all those small clothes over all those years, I would jinx myself and never lose any weight. I did finally get rid of a ton of clothes and all those small sizes. They were given away to churches, Goodwill, consignment shops, and women's shelters. Little did I know that I should have kept a few of those smaller sizes for the following year when I shrunk after my health transformation.

The big front office right off the front door in the old house was okay when I was alone, but not when Dave was home with me and that was another reason why I was excited to move into the new house. I worked from home for over a decade, and Dave and I really got along well together, except after golf. Dave would come home from golf about two in the afternoon, and of course promptly have a nap. My big front office right off the front hallway did not have any doors. It was an oversized opening and we investigated many different ways to enclose it with a new frame and door but never got around to doing anything. When Dave came home from golf, and if I had a virtual demo or a conference call planned in the afternoon, I had to put this sign up on the garage door:

"No Snoring, No Burping, No Farting, No Flushing of the toilet – DEMO IN PROGRESS!"

It didn't really work though, because that nap was the number one priority for Dave, and of course he couldn't control his snoring lying in the recliner on his back. I forgive you, Dave, really. I was happy the new house had an office in the back with a door I could close! About the snoring—after his brain aneurysm and the craniotomy, he magically stopped snoring in bed. Not a recommended solution, but a nice side effect.

It was a rough summer getting ready to move. Dave was a bear and very emotional. Those two months were busy and very stressful on top of it, between fixing the old house up, painting, and getting rid of fifteen years of stuff. Oracle kept me busy at work on top of it, traveling and helping lead business deals in my role on the application software sales side. Dave may have not known himself why he was feeling this way, but he didn't feel well, he was cranky, and he was not sleeping well.

Dave actually went back on the road once we signed the deal to buy Deb's house, to start selling his personal supply of tools. He had a blast visiting and selling to service stations around Charleston just like the old days when he was a firefighter and selling Makita Power tools as a side business. Dave had a very successful business selling these tools. (Most firefighters had side jobs because of their unusual 28 day calendar shift work.) He had kept and accumulated lots of tools in his stash in the garage. This is another reason I feel sure he must have known something was wrong.

Walking through the uncluttered garage after we learned the diagnosis and all the boxes had been unpacked, I would turn to Dave often and say, "You knew you were sick, didn't you?" He always told me no, but I wasn't convinced. There were boxes that we hadn't unpacked from the other house, from books to record albums to old camping gear. They were all gone.

Dear friend Cyndy that month came up with an idea for Dave's Cobalt Blue glass collection. These were pieces he had from his family like an old apothecary bottle, and some antiques he collected for himself. There were also pieces we bought on our travels, like the blue fish and sailboat from Hawaii and a special double candle holder piece from Venice of blown glass (airport security thought it looked like a gun!). Some were gifts from friends, and others were presents I found from all over. He was so sad that our glass table with the blue glass collection on it from the old house wouldn't fit anywhere in the new house, and he said with a long face, "It's okay, it doesn't matter." Yeah right, I knew he didn't mean it!

Ms. Cyndy said something to me that I'll never forget, "When guys have and collect sh#$, you gotta put it out," so we did. Dave left for golf one day and Cyndy and I unpacked all the blue glass, storing away the boring crystal bowl collection that was there, and filled the dining room hutch with his prized collection. The look on his face when he came home from golf and saw our surprise of his prized collection displayed prominently in the dining room is burned in my memory. It first brought a look of frozen shock on his face while he processed what he was seeing and quickly turned to happiness and love when he realized what we did for him. This moment was absolutely priceless for not only me, but Cyndy too.

Life had been so frantic since that day at the gym in June with Deb. After we finally moved all the boxes into the house mid-September, it took until October to get totally unpacked. I remember sitting in the sunroom and saying to Dave, "We did it! We can finally relax and watch a movie."

Two weeks later, our friends Mark and Laura came in from Phoenix to visit us in Charleston, our first house guests in the new place. The day after they left, October 23, is another memorable date I'll never forget. I was reading the newspaper in the sunroom. Dave had gone to sleep early which was not normal, and he came out about 10:00 p.m. and said, "Sweetie, you need to take me to the hospital, because I think I'm having a heart attack."

"Not a chance I'm driving you to the hospital. We're calling an ambulance," I responded. He said, "No, I think I'm okay, but I need to get to the hospital." I trusted his firefighter training. We went to the Emergency Room yet again, and after many tests and many hours lying around, they found no evidence of a heart attack. They have a blood test that they do that tells you if you're having a heart attack or not, and it came back negative. I suspect it was pain from his not being able to swallow properly which had been occurring more often than not at that time.

That night began his last journey and his life's final battle.

When I think back over that year, Dave was having difficulty swallowing for a while and he used to say to me it felt like "the food got stuck." It got more and more difficult for Dave to swallow after that visit to the ER in October. The first stop after the hospital visit was to see Dave's primary doctor. He said to go get an endoscopy. It's probably nothing more than needing your esophagus stretched. And while you're at it, have a colonoscopy since it's the same doctor, but different ends. His doctor texted his friend the gastroenterologist and got Dave in for a consultation. The actual endoscopy and colonoscopy didn't get scheduled after this until the end of November. My role as a caregiver during our time together meant never leaving him alone, so I was with Dave when he came out of anesthesia a LOT of times, and it took him an extra-long time to come around this time. This was unusual and I was a little scared, as it normally took him no time at all to come around. The first thing he said to me when he woke up was, "Honey, I don't feel any relief when I swallow."

The doctor came in a few minutes later and said the first words that began the doom and gloom roller coaster ride of emotions, "You have a tumor." He texted his friend the surgeon, and off we went down that path hoping the tumor could be cut out. The first test he scheduled was a CT scan. Why he just didn't order a PET scan at that point, I don't know. Only that type of scan would confirm the tumor in the esophagus was cancerous.

Dr. Google told me that.

The scan lit up like a Christmas tree, and we learned it was cancer—stage four. Not just in the tumor in his esophagus, but now it spread to his liver, lungs, and stomach. They gave it a name; it was esophageal cancer.

After we got the news, the next step was to visit the oncologist. We did this before Christmas and before we learned of the prognosis. The protocol they suggested was a brutal one, with lots of extreme side effects such as having to wear gloves if you opened the refrigerator, loss of taste, nausea of course, and many more they told us about that day. It's a nasty cocktail of medications, and we did a lot of research. Dave told the oncologist he'd think about each option and give him the final decision after the holidays.

Four brain surgeries, two hip replacements, and two knee replacements—again—was it any wonder when the cancer diagnosis came we thought he'd beat it no problem?

We'd been going away for Christmas since about 2010 and we had our timeshare condo already booked for Florida. We decided to leave town anyway even after the diagnosis. People told me NOT to google the survival rates of esophageal cancer, but of course I did. I never shared the bleak news from what I learned with Dave though, because it was not good. I was confident he didn't google the same thing (the only purpose for him having an iPad was to play solitaire, watch YouTube videos on how to fix stuff, and read his library books).

Heading south, after the PT scans, MRIs, CT scans, and visits with all the various doctors, we knew then the prognosis wasn't good. Dave really wanted to spend as much time as possible with our dear friend Debbie who lived in Orlando and had been with me every step of the way since the first test; we shared every result and every emotion imaginable. Her heart sank when she first learned of Dave's diagnosis.

It was the same cancer her beloved Ken passed away from a short time before. She would say to us, Ken didn't die the day we put him in the ground, he died the day he started chemo. This resonated with Dave; if there wasn't hope for a cure, why go through the agony of chemo?

We left for Florida with heavy minds and hearts. The news of this latest health scare was sinking in slowly, but we were ready to fight for life. After all, look at what he already survived so far in just one lifetime.

Dave loved his hockey, and we managed to get tickets to a Tampa game with Debbie along with a room at the Marriott Waterfront right across the street from Amalie Stadium. It was a good night, our first night in Florida, and we enjoyed the delicious buffet at Fire Stick inside the rink. Dave happened to put some raw oysters from the raw bar on his plate and Debbie and I looked at each other and said simultaneously, "NO! Don't eat those!" We both knew if you're immunocompromised, you shouldn't eat raw seafood.

The next day was pretty special. We went to Ybor City on the Trolley, enjoyed a Cuban coffee and a Sweet Lips cigar. It was as if we had to enjoy every single minute of our time left together on earth. It was emotional and sweet. The outpouring of love between us grew more and more frequent.

The hugs that week were more intense than ever.

Christmas Eve that year was quite sad. How do you buy a present for someone whose life is coming to an end? The picture I have of me and Dave with Santa at our condo in Florida is just priceless. He made me sit in Santa's lap and the smile on his face was great—like a little kid! I remember thinking how meaningless "stuff" was and my only secret wish for Santa was to have and hold Dave as long as I could.

On Christmas Day, we went to the Ritz Carlton for dinner at the Highball and Harvest restaurant which was excellent. Laughing and singing and dancing like nothing was wrong and our future was bright! Dave even came out singing after his visit to the restroom, joining in with the carolers in the lobby which I have a video of and love to listen to when I want to hear his voice. He couldn't eat much, but his spirits were good and his positivity apparent. Was he just putting on a brave face for me on our last Christmas? I think so now, but I'll never know for sure.

During those two weeks in Florida, we talked about everything under the sun. He really wanted to cross the t's and dot the i's for the million little details to make sure my path was set as well as his. Things like wills, cars, passwords, houses, deeds, bank accounts, just to name a few.

Nearing the end of our stay in Orlando, I asked, "Honey, where do you want to go, do you want to stay here or go somewhere else?" And he said, "I need to see the ocean and walk on the beach."

I must say I think I've spent one half of my life booking travel, whether it was for work, play, cruises or for our road trips. This time, I managed to book a last-minute oceanfront room at the Hilton in Daytona Beach, and when we arrived, Dave, as usual, was in charge of the luggage, valet, and parking the truck while I checked in. I was negotiating with the beautiful agent at the front desk on the type of rooms available for an upgrade. She showed me a few options, and when we returned to the front desk, she said to me, "Just wait a minute." She went to the back office and talked to the manager. She came out and said, "The Presidential Suite is available, but it's way more than what I quoted you." I quickly replied and said, "It doesn't matter, just do me a favor and don't put the bill under the door in the morning. I don't want Dave to see it."

I'll never forget the look of awe on Dave's face when we walked into the palatial Presidential Suite. It was perfect because when we got married at the Radisson in Niagara Falls, we had the presidential suite then too. But we didn't get to enjoy it because our wedding party totally trashed the room. It was covered with silly string, beds were short sheeted and covered with marbles, and there was toilet paper wrapped around everything! We ended up renting another room just to get some sleep that night. That is why this Presidential Suite was absolutely perfect. It had a huge terrace overlooking the ocean where we sat and had cocktails while watching the ocean. I've got some wonderful videos of Dave singing and talking to me on the balcony from that trip—more memories to relive.

There were sad memories as well. One night I wanted to create a video of him speaking to me as a keepsake, and he poured out his love for me, our life together, and he ended the recording with, "You know I love you so much." This chokes me up as I write this, and when I listen to the replay, I'm so thankful I have this keepsake.

We spent two magical nights there and came home to a shocking dose of reality that shook us to the core.

When we got home, there were at least fifteen messages on the phone. The oncologist had gone ahead, without our approval, and booked an appointment to have the port installed in Dave's chest for the chemo treatments. There were preparation messages for chemo, there was blood work to be done, more testing to be scheduled, and of course the financial department of the hospital wanted to make sure we could pay.

At this point, we hadn't even told the oncologist what our decision was yet. Panic set in, taking over the grounded calmness we felt from those two weeks in Florida. We were able to find some peace there, the weather had been perfect, and we felt strong to tackle the next step, or whatever else that might be in store for us.

As we drove to the oncologist that afternoon for a two o'clock appointment, it felt like we were going to a funeral, both of us filled with doom and gloom. When we arrived, we were very somber and in shock, walking slowly hand-in-hand into the office. The waiting room at the cancer center was also where the chemo patients came and checked in and it had the "bell" which the patients rang when they had their last chemo treatment.

The first question we asked the oncologist doctor was, "What's the prognosis?" The second question was if Dave was a candidate for immunotherapy (he wasn't), and what's the best guess? The doctor told us six months without chemo. We then asked the magic question: How long with chemo? And he said, "Maybe six months more." Dave knew that if there wasn't a chance for a cure, he wasn't going to go through with chemo treatments.

Dave replied, "No thank you, I'm going to opt for quality of life rather than quantity." He never for one second regretted that decision, he knew the side effects of chemo were horrific, and I feel at peace that he made this decision totally on his own. We never saw the oncologist again after that day. After all, he was only around for one reason—the very lucrative chemotherapy treatments. The doctor did try to persuade us with a few more weak arguments, but none addressing quality of life or a cure which was what Dave was after. A lot of friends and family questioned him after he made this decision, and the answer was the same, quality of life was the key for him. I feel good that he made the decision entirely on his own. Not once did he ask me what I thought; he was that sure of the path he had chosen and never questioned himself.

Not many go this route of saying "no" to chemo. I think it's tied to the "Doctor is God" theory; most people follow their doctor's advice blindly and without question.

We received a copy of a book from a friend and neighbor, Mary Ellen, called, *Being Mortal: Medicine and What Matters in the End* written by surgeon Atul Gawande. The book was very painful and emotional to read, but both of us got through it in the following months, many times in tears. It addressed the doctor's belief that quality of life should be the desired goal, not quantity. The surgeon explored hospice care to show a person's last weeks and months may be rich and dignified and this described Dave perfectly, right up to the minute he died. We were so glad we read the book; it was affirmation that he made the right decision, not that Dave needed it.

There was a peace and love between us which would not be shaken.

For the next four months, Dave woke up every morning and said two things, "Good morning, beautiful" and "I feel terrific!" He was in really good spirits and feeling okay until the last couple weeks on earth.

I often wonder about the unusual weather that year. We got a snowstorm that shut down our southern city for four days. There wasn't a lot of snowfall, but in the south there's no salt, snow removal equipment, or four-wheel drive vehicles. It was freezing for the whole month of January and February and March. I think back now and wonder if it was the universe helping out so Dave didn't miss his weekly golf too much.

My health insurance benefits at the time included a second opinion for cancer screening. We flew to New York City and went to Sloan Kettering. We went through a half a day of tests, never seeing the oncologist doctor, but two days later she called us with her opinion. She said, "You must have chemo. We must shrink the tumor," and we both said, "But for what?" She said with animated emotion in her voice, "So you can eat!" She was shocked that Dave wouldn't take her advice. After all, even if they did shrink the tumor so that food could pass, he wouldn't feel like eating anyway because of the horrific side effects. He was so brave and stuck by his convictions. Chemo destroys your appetite and ability to eat, so what difference would that make if the tumor was smaller? Everyone said chemo, chemo, chemo.

Everyone except Dave.

CHAPTER 4

Hot Times at the Firehouse

"When I think of Dave, I think of three words that start with a capital P: Passion, Perseverance, and Profanity."

This was how Chief Al Hills kicked off not only the 1st Dave Scott Memorial Golf Tournament in 2018, but also when he came back for the 2nd Annual Memorial the next year. The crowd roared, and everyone there who knew Dave laughed because it was so true. I personally can vouch for all three words: Passion, Perseverance, and Profanity. Dave had passion for everything he did, from his ski patrol years helping "haul wrecks" off the ski hill as he called it, to our love and life together, to his golf game, and most of all to his career as a firefighter and then rising to Captain. Keeping his men safe above all else was the most important thing to him. Dave showed perseverance in everything he attempted, from getting me to go out to dinner with him after we met at Gray Rocks, to breaking ninety on the golf course, to learning how to do just about everything around the house from his numerous "how-to" books and later from YouTube videos. He dabbled in electricity, plumbing, all kinds of repairs, landscaping for all the different climates we lived in, and fixing his truck. The profanity—well, let's just say it was frequent and mostly came out for the little stuff that happened in life, like missing a putt, screwing his thumb to the wall while hanging a picture in my office, hitting his thumb with a hammer, or slicing a golf drive. The profanity was always right on the tip of his tongue. In fact, when we golfed with Terry, who didn't ever swear, if she had a bad golf shot, she'd say, "Dadgummit, and all the bad words Dave knows!" The profanity never came out for the big crises, like the basement flooding, almost cutting his finger off, or stopping for an accident we may have come across on the road (and he ALWAYS stopped to lend a helping hand). His little blue ski patrol first aid kit was always with him in the truck, and it came in handy many times. My Mom had a saying, "Don't sweat the small stuff," but Dave always sweated the small stuff.

My perspective on his career is when you are constantly dealing with life, death, and destruction, it makes a firefighter a special person. The many incidents Dave was a part of all affected him deeply. There were tragedies like the nursing home fire, train wrecks which caused the largest evacuation in Canada, a parking garage ceiling collapse, and babies dying in his arms. Full of caring, empathy, and with a unique perspective on life, Dave carried this with him right to the end.

Dave serving and being a firefighter with his single-minded purpose to help others shaped me and my career. He was my best life and career coach and helped make me into the woman I am today. It's nice to have a man like that to have your back and support some of your crazy dreams, and he loved to help me with my college homework.

Chief Al joined Dave's crew as a rookie and then rose to Platoon Chief over his thirty-year career. Al's speech before dinner at the Golf Memorial talked about occupational illnesses, like cancer, becoming greater than the incidents of safety deaths for firefighters. This was because of the many strides the fire service made over the years to prevent deadly incidents and accidents. January is now designated as the Fire Fighter Cancer Awareness Month, as it's that serious of an issue for firefighters. The connection between different kinds of cancer and firefighters was and is real. Between the smoke inhalation, to the toxins in burning fires, to unhealthy habits like washing smoky clothes at home, the links to cancer-causing agents and routines are numerous. There is also a big push for wellness programs in the departments today, learning about nutrition and detoxification needed to prevent this cancer rise.

Chief Al Hills procured a special "MSA Fire Helmet" as a raffle giveaway for the golf memorial tournament. He wrote this note and attached it for the donation:

"Captain Dave Scott worked for thirty years at Mississauga Fire & Emergency Services (outside of Toronto, Ontario) in a City of 700,000 residents. His dedication to the citizens and to his crew members was unparalleled. In the spirit of Captain Dave Scott, MSA (a large fire protection company in Pittsburgh) has donated a yellow Cairns Fire Captain helmet; the type that was used by Dave during his firefighting duties. Firefighters wear black helmets and Captains wear yellow helmets in Mississauga to distinguish the officer in charge at the emergency scene."

When the helmet went up for auction, it raised $500 more for the Youth Hockey Scholarship fund. The next time I saw that helmet it brought tears to my eyes, again. My friend Patty bought it, and I did not know the reason why until we went there for their awesome annual Christmas party. She brought me out to the garage, and there on the wall was her grandfather's fire helmet from the '30s, her brother's helmet, and Dave's yellow Captain's helmet, all occupying spots of honor on the wall. Her grandmother was also a matron at the firehouse. What a collection of stories hanging on that wall.

Dave was laser focused on safety for his men. Even after he retired, he always ended his emails or calls or greetings with "stay safe" and for me, every time I flew, he'd call and say, "fly safe." It was funny; if he realized he forgot to tell me, he'd call me back immediately just to tell me to "fly safe!"

Fire halls, stations, houses, firehouses—what's the difference? Dave used to simply call it the "station." I had a lot of input from people in the know on where these different terms came from. The time I spent talking with firefighters at the Line of Duty Deaths Memorial Ceremonies in Ottawa, Colorado Springs, and Toronto helped clarify the answer to the different names. For example, the New Yorkers called them simply "houses." According to Chief Al Hills, the term "fire stations" is a very Canadian term. He thought the most appropriate term for the book to be widely recognized would be "firehouse." Finally, Mike, a retired firefighter and neighbor I met golfing in a tournament, clearly outlined the difference. He shared that "Firehall" was the common term for volunteer departments. The reason was they often rented out the halls for parties so that's why they called them "fire halls." I took Al's advice and changed the title!

The esophageal cancer Dave had was considered one of fourteen "presumptive" cancers, commonly called "Firefighter's Cancer." Because of this, he was honored as a Line of Duty Death (LODD) through the IAFF, International Association of Firefighters. When Dave started his career, they didn't wear masks. Breathing apparatus came many years later. Dave actually started the application for this recognition leading to the LODD designation, back in January after his diagnosis, with the urging of our dear friend Sue.

Dave was accepted as a Line of Duty Death (LODD) after he died. Because of this, it meant LODD ceremonies in three places – Ottawa, Colorado Springs, and Toronto. I learned at those ceremonies that most of the men engraved on the walls died from occupational illnesses, not firefighter accidents. Dave would be so honored and proud to know his name is forever etched on these three walls.

Al Hills told me about some of the recent safety changes for the better, especially in the arena of environmental toxins that have come about since Dave retired. The men no longer took their fire gear home to wash; some of the toxins they were exposed to would never leave the washer and perhaps get mixed in with the baby clothes in the next wash. They now have washers and dryers in every firehouse. I'll never forget finding this funny looking hood in the laundry one time; I had no clue what it was. I was worried Dave had taken to robbing banks because I was on the road for work so much! It turned out to be his Nonex fire hood. That was the first and last time he brought gear home, because the rules changed about bringing stuff home to wash shortly thereafter.

YOUR MOTHER DOESN'T LIVE HERE!

That was the sign above the kitchen sink at the Lakeview Firehouse in Mississauga where Dave spent many years as Captain. One of my favorite sayings over the years was "Firefighters make great wives." I always told everyone that because they cook, clean, do toilets, windows, cry at sad movies (or the National Anthem for that matter!); they just know how to do it all with a sense of service, humor, and sensitivity. Dave did all that and more. All the things they experienced from fire destruction—horrific accidents where they had to use the jaws of life, lots of medical calls, and saving lives—contributed to firefighters being so sensitive. Their WICKED sense of humor coupled with living so closely together in the firehouse made for some hilarious stories.

My first experience with this always present sense of humor was at our wedding in Niagara Falls. We were all sitting at the bar before the rehearsal dinner and I remember Firefighter Bill, who was on Dave's crew, turning to my Dad and asking, "Who are you?" Dad says proudly, "I'm giving away the bride." Without one second's hesitation Bill says, "I hope you got a good price!" Next, the fire alarms were set off that night and the sprinklers came on at the hotel we were staying at for our wedding. The guys were standing around outside and they said to Dave, "Nice job getting the trucks here. How did you pull that one off?!" The sprinklers ruined my handwritten place settings (I did calligraphy back then), but it didn't matter. It was priceless and a perfect memory to have from that weekend. Of course, all the firefighters on Dave's crew were hanging around the truck looking at the equipment like kids in a candy store.

Fellow firefighter Errol told me about a couple of pranks they pulled on Dave while working at headquarters. One of the best was when they put Dave's car, rear end up, on blocks, not realizing he had one of the first front wheel drive cars. So he easily drove off the blocks laughing at the guys over his shoulder.

Dave told this story for years about a phone booth next to a bus stop below HQ's big floor to ceiling glass windows overlooking the street. Joe Shaw got the number to that phone, and when someone would walk by, he'd ring the booth and ask them to clap their hands to check the volume! I think the firefighters had nothing on Candid Camera.

The guys would kill themselves laughing behind those big windows at headquarters. Camaraderie, laughter, family, his men, friends—Dave cherished it all.

Another time, the Post Office cemented a post box on a wall across the street from HQ. The firehouse guys posted a sign above the closed box which said, "Push the fourth brick over four rows up" so they could watch what happened through those big windows. They thought nobody would fall for it, but a few did! The funniest was when a young guy wearing a University of Toronto jacket walked up to the wall and read the note. They all cracked up laughing, watching him count the bricks and push the fourth one over. Simple delights for those long shifts. The firehouse was really their second home. All the men were quite close; it truly was a brotherhood.

The Christmas incident is legendary and I heard Dave tell this funny story every single year we were together. It was at Christmas time, and one of the guys found a box of music chips like they put in musical greeting cards, and the song was "Jingle Bells" on every single chip in the box. The guys (yes, all guys; women came into the department much later) put one in the ceiling vent in Dave's office/

bedroom and it turned him into a raving lunatic. He couldn't figure out where it was coming from. When he finally found it, he thought, now what can I do with the rest of these music chips to get the guys back? He ended up putting one in a rookie's car, and every time the car started, "Jingle Bells" would play. I don't remember how long it took him to figure out where it was coming from.

Dave had the best and greatest laugh. I can still hear it in reliving and retelling these stories in this book. (I often told Dave HE should have written a book with all his firehouse stories.) It was such a key to the type of men in the firehouses.

Every firefighter had a nickname; it was required—the first thing issued right after the equipment. Paul Flakt was Nurse; Steve Stone was Stoney; Albert was Dave's; Nudle belonged to Bob Doddridge; Gord Key was Gordie. The nicknames were funny and every single one had to be different. "Scary," AKA Mike Scarangella, told me about a time when they hired someone with a similar last name to his and the guys in that firehouse wanted to nickname him "Scary" and it was immediately rejected because there was already a Scary! Bill Campbell was "Soupy." This one still makes me laugh every time I hear it. Errol was Frenchy because he lived in Quebec for a while, Fred LeBlac was Budder, and his Dad was called "Bud." It was a special community of good men who were very close in so many ways.

Sundays at the firehouse meant one of the men (they rotated each week) had to buy, cook, and feed six to ten hungry men. These Sunday breakfasts were the original definition of "supersized" meals. When it was Dave's turn for breakfast, it meant buying two loaves of bread, two dozen eggs, five pounds of bacon, and the mandatory baked beans. Yes, baked beans for breakfast.

My brother Mike had an interesting observation while we were at the Colorado Springs Line of Duty Death ceremony. He said, "Every single firefighter falls into two categories, either they're "jacked" (super fit calendar material), or they have a belly." I looked around at the 2,500 volunteer firefighters there from all over the US and Canada, and he was right! Dave was in the latter category. Desserts for Dave meant two scoops of ice cream. He could not resist dessert. And there were a lot of midnight snacks eaten over his thirty-year career.

I learned later about the tie between sugar and cancer which is not good. Sugar feeds cancer cells. I tried to always send Dave to work with homecooked leftover meals. We tried to eat healthy and I tried to cook healthy meals, but it wasn't enough. There were the temptations at the firehouse and temptations we couldn't resist when we ate out at a restaurant, and that was often.

Dennis (a.k.a. Denny O') O'Rafferty shared this funny story with me, a story I hadn't heard before. He told me, "You know Davy struggled with his weight. Well, he would go into the upstairs dorm, put on his tights, draw the drapes, and put on his "Dancersize" music. That's when the four of us, Glennie, Stevie, Billy, and myself would climb the TV antenna tower and try every possible way to catch a glimpse of Captain Dave Scott exercising in his tights. When he saw us this one time, we knew we were busted. He threw open the drapes and there we were laughing our asses off. But you know Dave, he always got the last laugh. So, he says, you want to have some ladder practice, do you? That was our punishment, taking ladders on and off trucks all day long! We all laughed for years about this."

Dennis ended the story with, "God bless my old friend. He now has the body he always wanted."

9/11 was a traumatic and gut-wrenching time for every firefighter watching those towers fall, and Dave was no exception. We were living in Northern Virginia at the time where I had been relocated to from Rochester, NY. I was between jobs because of the "dot-com" bubble which burst, causing layoffs all over the tech sector. Dave was a jack of all trades, and he was helping our dear friend Marv renovate his garage while I was busy looking for another job.

The morning of 9/11, as usual, the TV was tuned to CNBC. Dave was a stock market fanatic, always studying companies and stocks and carefully investing for us and our future. When the first tower got hit, I was thinking, okay, it was just a crazy accident. As a frequent flyer my whole life, when the second tower got hit, I knew something was up; there's no way both could be a fluke incident. Next to be hit was the Pentagon, only thirty minutes away from our townhouse. They closed down the state of Virginia shortly after that, and the government shut down after the Pentagon incident. Dave immediately came flying home in his truck from our friend Marv's house where he was helping with a large garage project. The biggest fear we had, being so close to the Pentagon, was fear of the unknown. Who was doing this and what was next; the world was on edge and we were, too. From our balcony in the townhouse, we would hear and watch the fighter jets flying circles around the city, and we would tense up when we heard the roar.

When we watched the towers fall later that morning, he was devastated and in tears. He couldn't move off the couch for three days, glued to the television. Every single firefighter watching knew that all the men were climbing UP to rescue everyone, and they weren't going to make it back down. Visiting NYC was very hard for Dave after 9/11. We did go one time to the memorial and walked by the firehouse (Ten House) that lost so many men. I could see Dave trembling as we got nearer.

We were living outside of Charleston, South Carolina, when the tragic Charleston Nine Sofa Super Store fire occurred back in 2007. That fire ranked next in the highest number of firefighter fatalities in a single event since 9/11. It was a serious fire in Charleston, and Dave couldn't even bring himself to read the report. The fatalities could have been prevented with modern safety regulations which had been implemented years before in Canada. Some of the faults included ineffective on-scene incident command and inadequate equipment used by the department that evening. Dave was beside himself, especially as a captain, because he knew he held his men's lives in his hands. This was another reason why Dave and crew did training every single shift so they all remained current and sharp.

Dave's favorite saying, that had to have come from the fire department because of the toughness they dealt with, was "You know where you can find sympathy? Between shit and syphilis in the dictionary." Another favorite saying, also I think because of all the death and suffering he'd seen in his job, was, "You're a long time dead." We never hesitated doing anything or saving things for after I retired. Except for getting a dog; he said when he retired, we'd get a dog, along with a cat for me. I had a cat when we met, Darius the Persian. Darius the cat loved to snuggle in Dave's hairy armpits like he was sniffing catnip, purring away like crazy.

Dave's uniform every single day (well, other than golf days!) since he retired was a blue "job" shirt which he collected from firehouses on our travels. Every city we went to, the first stop was the firehouse to buy a T-shirt. Most of the time, the captain on shift would kindly just give Dave a shirt. Needless to say, every single one of his T-shirts told a story. The only place we failed to get a T-Shirt was in Florence, Italy. Dave spotted a fire truck on the streets and tried to engage the Italian crew in conversation, but it didn't work! They just smiled and drove on.

No matter where we traveled, Dave had brothers in firehouses around the world.

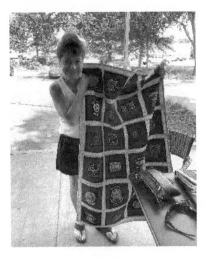

We put many of his favorite T Shirts on display hanging in the pavilion at the 1st annual Golf Memorial, but for the 2nd Golf Memorial, they were displayed in two beautiful "forever quilts." We started by cutting out the firehouse logos on my dining room table under the watchful eye of my friend Cyndy, a Master Quilter. We had enough left over for a second, smaller quilt. More treasured memories to hold and be wrapped up in forever.

If those firehouse T-shirts could talk, what stories they'd tell. The IAFF international union crest is very recognizable. Every time I see the crest when I'm out walking, if it's on a blue T-shirt, I do a double take, my mind thinking it's Dave back by my side.

The Batcave FDNY station twenty-six has that name because it's really hard to find. The Bat Cave is on 38th and 7th in NYC. We did find it though, and the funniest scene greeted us. Two firefighters were putting tie straps around a foot high Batman on the front grill of the fire truck. Apparently, it got stolen so much, they thought this method (other than chaining it to the firetruck grill), would let them keep it a little bit longer. We visited many NYC firehouses, including: Rescue 1 midtown 43rd and 10th, Pride engine 54 at 48th and 8th, and Engine Six. We loved New York City, and T-shirts from there were his favorite ones to wear.

The city that never sleeps is a perfect description; we enjoyed every visit. From Broadway to the Italian restaurants to the nightlife and music in Greenwich Village to the wonderful hotels to Katz's deli for corned beef stacked high (especially if you tipped a dollar!)—we loved a lot of different things about NYC.

Daytona Beach was a funny T-shirt story. We showed up at the firehouse on the water, and no one was there. We called the number on the door, and the City Commissioner actually drove out and opened up the hall just to get Dave a T-shirt. Yes, it's that important.

I had a hand in the Honolulu T-shirt for a surprise Christmas present. It was Christmas Eve, and I decided to venture out and find the firehouse in Honolulu. It took a while. After two separate buses and a taxi, it kind of reminded me of my trip trying to get to Gray Rocks where we first met. This was before I was an Uber customer. You should've seen Dave's face the next morning on Christmas day when he opened up the T-shirt. It was the best gift ever, in his eyes.

With amazing zest for life, Dave invited and sought out adventures wherever he went if he was with me on work travels or if we were on vacation together. One of his first stops would always be the local firehouse for coffee, a T-shirt of course, and insider tips on where to eat and what to do. The Denver T-shirt was especially memorable to him. I was working, he was traveling with me, and he found the firehouse and stopped in for a cup of coffee. Firehouses ALWAYS had the coffee on. The Chief on duty put some papers in front of him and said, "Sign here." Dave had no idea what was about to happen, but he signed the forms, and the Chief said, "Get in the truck." They proceeded to spend the day together on the streets of Denver. He had an amazing day and was just bursting like a kid to tell me all about it when we connected for cocktails and dinner that night after my work day.

The Boston T-shirts hold a great memory. I was in Boston for a team meeting which I organized. Event planning was a love of mine, and I was thankful Oracle let me raise my hand to volunteer. I planned some exciting meetings over the years. Boston was exciting and by far the best. I actually arranged batting practice with the Red Sox under the Green Monster wall at Fenway with the help of my neighbor and rabid Red Sox fan, Kevin. Needless to say, Dave was *so* jealous! I ended up flying him out after the team meeting, and I got tickets to another game and a private tour of Fenway. We visited two firehouses that trip and came home with new T-shirts for his private collection. He was so happy to get a shirt from the hall who called themselves "First into Fenway," the famous baseball stadium of the Red Sox.

The Colorado Springs T-shirt is especially poignant when I look at that logo from his collection, now on the quilt. Dave's name was written on the Colorado Spring LODD wall on September 21, 2019. I remembered one trip to Colorado Springs; I was there on a project, and Dave was with me. We found the National firefighters Memorial purely by accident wandering around the city, and it brought tears to his eyes when he saw some firefighters' names from his town of Mississauga and from all over Canada etched on the wall. This was the first memorial we ever saw, not realizing these were all over the world.

He never dreamed his name would one day be among those men honored.

The first of three ceremonies was held in Ottawa. Bob and Georgette Bogle drove down from outside Kingston, Ontario, to be by my side. The Bogles were our friends who we met in 1998 while golfing in Rochester, and we remained good friends despite moving farther and farther away from each other over the years.

Chief Al Hills and his beautiful wife Linda joined us as well. Al began as a rookie on Dave's crew, and rose to be Platoon Chief of Mississauga.

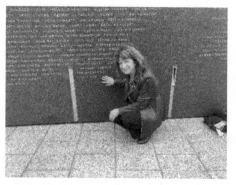

Driving in my taxi from the airport to the Sheraton hotel in Ottawa, I was overcome with emotion, thinking about what this would have meant to Dave. I arrived at the hotel, in tears, not knowing what to expect, but I didn't have to worry for a second. As soon as I registered, I wasn't alone at any time during those three days. The support of the Fallen Firefighters group was amazing, every single step of the way.

I'm so glad I went to Ottawa before attending the huge International (US and Canada) ceremony in Colorado Springs. Colorado Springs was incredible and overwhelming, with over 2,500 volunteers there from the fire departments across the US and Canada. Dear friends Peter and Maryann from Phoenix were also by my side, along with my brothers Rich and Mike from Rochester, and friends Laura and Mark from Phoenix. I was honored with a presentation of the IAFF flag during the ceremony. Laura turned to me at the Colorado Springs ceremony and said, "There's only one person who would have had more fun being here." I was puzzled and said, "Who?" She said "Dave!!" I laughed, because he loved a party, loved his fire department career, loved his men, and loved his friends.

He'd be talking up a storm with everyone, and I can envision him laughing and telling stories, doing shots of Jameison whiskey, and of course, he'd be collecting every single one of the T-shirts they had on display in the tents.

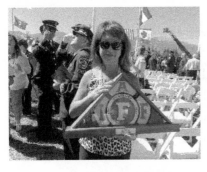

Colorado Springs was amazing in many ways. My two brothers joined me, coincidentally with a plane full of firefighters from New York going to recognize some of their men who had fallen and whose names would be etched into the wall. They were still losing men from 9/11 from lingering illnesses along with other occupational illnesses.

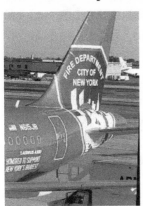

My brother's flight the night before was cancelled, so they were delayed until the next day. As they were going through JFK to catch their connection, they spotted this plane with the tail decorated to honor the Fire Department of New York, and they took a picture to send to me. I was already in Denver. Little did they know, they were getting ON that plane. Almost 95% of the flight was made up of firefighters, and they had a blast. The stories from that flight! The Captain got on the speaker and made an announcement "I'm sorry, the plane has run out of alcohol." It was only ten in the morning. Brother Mike was sitting in a middle seat next to a firefighter who apparently had a tough shift, and then later it was understood that he went out the night before which is why he was passed out and drooling. Of course, his fellow firefighters were laughing themselves silly and taking pictures from all angles. I'm sure he'll never live that down.

Brother Rich was sitting in the back by the bathroom and he

described the scene like being in a bar with a constant stream of firefighters in the aisles, giving big manly hugs to everyone, cursing up a storm, and using the toilet. What a fitting flight cancellation it was for them, setting the stage for the next five days we'd be together in Colorado Springs.

Thousands of volunteers were involved in the motorcycle procession that started the day and operating the truck parade with equipment from all over the US and Canada. Even the bagpipe players in the streets were all volunteers. The videos of the volunteers playing the bagpipes gets me emotional every single time. Tears flowed the whole weekend. I will never forget the outpouring of support from every single avenue.

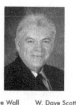

The picture of W. Dave Scott when he retired in 1998 and will be forever accessible through the IAFF (International Association of Firefighters) App on any mobile device. The picture is his official retirement photo. I have offered to volunteer at the Colorado Springs Memorial. It moved me so much that I was so well taken care of in such a time of

Name on the Wall	W. Dave Scott
Local Number	L1212
Local Name	Mississauga
Location on Wall	78
Date of Passing	April 15, 2018
Cause	Cancer · Esophageal

raging emotions that I want to help return the compassion to others in the same situation.

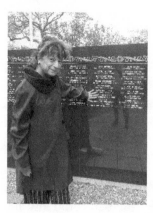

Toronto was the last ceremony, and the most moving and meaningful, because it was where Dave spent his entire thirty-year career. Bob and Sue Woodall joined me, along with Chief Al Hills and wife Linda. Here's the wall in Toronto.

RIP Captain Dave. You left the world a better place. You left many things better, including me, but the first year you were gone was the worst year of my life.

PART 2

The Middle

CHAPTER 5

Widowhood Wackiness— Firsts and Lasts

Widowhood sucks your brains out and leaves nothing behind but fog and dust and ashes sprinkled with a side of stupidity. I always said you need to surround yourself with smart friends because you're going to need them to get through your temporary incompetence. I love this saying: *A friend is a gift you give yourself.* So many friends helped me through the sad times, the grief, the early smiles (feeling *so* guilty), and the return from the dark shadows into the light again.

Speaking of ashes, Dave sent me a very loud message one day. I had a scattering tube of his ashes in his dresser armoire. One morning the door flew open, my jaw dropped, and I said, "I know, I know! I'll get right on the scattering!"

Grief is a many splendored thing. It can grab you by the neck and wrestle you to the ground in no time. It can also create incredibly good feelings when you lock yourself away reliving cherished memories of time spent with your favorite buddy. Dave and I were together for almost thirty years, falling short by only four months.

This thing called "widow fog" takes over your life. It's funny that after a whole life of being smart, efficient, organized, and an independent female road warrior, all of a sudden you're reduced to a puddle of babbling idiocy. I was making wrong travel plans, flying into the wrong cities, on the wrong dates, and having meltdowns in airports and planes all over the world.

Widow fog is a real scientific occurrence. My friend told me about widow's fog being tied to the prefrontal cortex of the brain, and it resonated. She pointed me to articles about the fog and the scientific reason why it's so real. That part of the brain is the part of the brain which handles rational thinking as well as making sense of your emotions. I interviewed a number of widows and widowers about situations they found themselves in under the guise of "widowhood brain fog." The stories they shared varied wildly, from mild to debilitating experiences from losing things like keys and cars, to not being able to get out of bed for days at a time.

There were a lot of what I called "stupid human tricks" that happened to me that first year. Some were funny, some were dangerous, and some were downright brain farts. I'll say again to my fellow widows and widowers: Surround yourself with smart friends who still have their brains; you're going to need help in that department. My friend Sue of thirty years flew down from Toronto for a week right after Dave died and helped me tremendously with all the legal paperwork for both the US and Canada. My friends and neighbors all rallied around to help supplement my lack of brain power in the early months. Some of my smart friends happened to be widows as well, like Linda, Debbie, Cyndy, Deb. So thankful to have had them around.

The stupidest and most dangerous thing I did early on was drive away from the gas station with the hose still in my car. As I pulled away from the pump, I knew immediately what I had done. I quickly looked in the side mirror expecting to see the gas station up in flames, just like in the movies. Thank goodness it didn't explode! The first thing my friends asked me was, "Did you scratch your new car?" No, I didn't scratch the car, and yes, I'm fine, thanks for asking! I've been driving for a really long time, decades in fact, and this was just a dumb thing to do. The good thing is it has made me paranoid every time I get gas now. I double and triple check my side mirror to make sure the pump is out of the tank. Almost as bad as walking back and forth to the house door over and over to double and triple check that the door is locked.

Still grief-struck and still numb with losing Dave, my dear Mom died in December of that same year. We really lost Mom mentally when Dad died in 2010; she withdrew into herself with her diagnosis of vascular dementia getting really bad. I happened to be with my friend Debbie in New York City over Thanksgiving weekend, the week before Mom died. I had to get to Rochester to see Mom, as she was in pretty bad shape, and I got a car to the airport to catch the flight I booked. The only problem with that was I left my license and credit cards at the hotel I was sharing with her. For some reason I had my passport with me which got me on the flights that day. Thank goodness Debbie was still there in our room, and she sent my license and credit cards overnight to the hotel I was staying at in Rochester. I felt like a novice traveler. This was something I had never done, ever. That wasn't a bad record for a person who has traveled for work and pleasure since I was seventeen years old.

Sometimes whole days were totally messed up from this all-consuming brain fog. I had my weekly gym visit scheduled with my trainer, Tyler, and drove halfway to the gym with the car hatch wide open. Since I was late (as usual), I mistakenly left the car running as I bolted inside the house to grab something, not realizing the hatch was still open. That's after dropping the phone on my eye that morning and cutting my forehead about three-quarters of an inch. It could've been worse—one more inch and I could've been blinded by my phone. I also sliced my finger that afternoon taking apart a big box. Stupid, dumbass day all the way around. To say that grief is distracting would be an understatement.

One fine Saturday morning in July (a short three months after Dave died), I had an early morning golf tee time with the girls. I got up at 5:15 a.m., stretched, packed an apple and some almonds, and ran out the door. Our golf course was really close, about a five-minute walk around the corner. About halfway up the block, I realized I didn't have golf shoes on, only my golf socks and no shoes at all. Back to the house I went. That was almost as silly as the day on my way to the gym when I put my sock on my hand instead of my foot, only shaved one leg, and had my shirt on inside out.

Have you ever gotten in the shower with your eyeglasses and socks still on? I have.

I had to stop and get cash and deposit a check at the ATM one Saturday. When the check wouldn't deposit because it was from Canada, I drove away from the ATM in a fuming huff. Off I went to find a parking spot, and then went storming into the branch to have a word with the manager about my Canadian check. The only problem was the bank card was still in the ATM machine, it hadn't spit it out yet, and I had to order a new one which took days! That made me feel pretty stupid.

The feeling of helplessness was overwhelming. Dave was weighing heavy on my mind. I was constantly losing something, or is it just misplaced when you find it days or weeks later? My keys, my glasses, my health care card, gift cards, my cash stash, my will, and loads of other things daily. Between feelings of despair, trying to function with work and dealing with the unpredictable throes of grief, my emotions were raging.

The brain fog did eventually lift, and I did find everything I lost, except for my will. I wasn't sure if my lawyer had a copy, but hopefully I won't need that for a while!

Widowhood does suck. The whole messy grieving process sucks. It's a club I never dreamed I'd be a part of. Grief has no timeline and no rulebook. Even after a few years for me, it's still right there, waiting to be called up to the surface with the tiniest triggers.

Things which brought back different memories popped up in the early months at the weirdest times and in the weirdest places. The photo album from our first year together appeared out of nowhere on my living room bookshelf. I have no idea how it got there. All the albums lived in the hutch in the dining room, always. It had pictures from our first date at Prince of Wales and the night we took our engagement pictures in Buffalo and came back to my house in Rochester.

Later that same week, as I was cleaning up the office, I came across Dave's little black book. He made the notation "Great Legs" by my name the night we met, December 6, 1986. This rose to the top, even after at least seven different house moves we had made.

Our last Valentine's Day was spent together at the club with our great group of friends and neighbors. For many, many years, our golf club put on a beautiful Valentine's Dinner. It was very romantic, beautifully decorated, with good service and good food, and we always enjoyed being with good friends and neighbors. The Valentine's Day card he bought me was the last card he ever gave to me. (That card would resurface a few years later on Valentine's Day morning as I was about to fly up to Maine to see my new boyfriend, Jeff. That is a whole other chapter in this book called "A Corona Love Story!")

I was washing blueberries at the sink one morning and started crying, remembering the last time Dave could get a blueberry down. He used to love a handful in his yogurt every single morning. And then I started thinking about coffee, and his last sip that final Saturday morning of his life. You loved your coffee, Dave, at least five or six cups a day.

I had to cancel the newspaper, along with canceling television out of my life. The stress of world events and the divisive climate of politics really took its toll on me. I remember Sachin Patel from the Living Proof Institute (after I began my health transformation) saying, "You can't do a thing about it, so tune it out." So, I did. In the old days, I'd be up from two to four o'clock in the morning watching the news. I'd scroll through the six news channels on my cable box. Once I stopped it really did reduce my stress level noticeably. Anxiety is tough enough to deal with on your own without having the weight of the world's problems on your shoulders. Grief and anxiety go hand in hand, worrying about the future without your right-hand man by your side.

Every day I rise and try to find something to smile about, thanks to my friend Deb. Deb is a widow as well, and one day I asked her how she got through her days. She is the one who told me, "I try to find something to smile about every single day," and that phrase stuck with me. Each morning I walk around the house, open all the blinds, try to stick my face in the sunlight, put the tea kettle on, and make myself my one cup of organic king coffee. Gratitude and thankfulness even for little things like a good cup of coffee, have the power to lessen grief I learned.

Dave and I loved to golf, a big reason why we lived in a golf course community. It took me a while to think about golfing again, but I knew it was a great way to meet people. A famous golf teacher once said, "There are no strangers on the golf course, only friends you haven't met yet." So I signed up for the World Amateur golf tournament in Myrtle Beach the following year after Dave died. My teammate Keith had talked about the World Am for years and said to me, "You have to come up and golf at this amazing event." I did finally sign up and went alone, joining 4,800 other golfers of all levels from around the world. (4,400 men and 400 women.) Going back solo to Myrtle Beach for the first time was quite emotional. Driving past the two hospitals Dave was admitted to for his brain aneurysm, driving past the golf courses we golfed at, and driving past Peter and Maryann's old neighborhood (which they left to move to Phoenix, AZ) brought back a ton of memories.

Walking on the beach the day before the tournament started, I came across a heart with the initials DS and MS etched in the sand, stopping me dead in my tracks. Dave Scott and Marie Scott. The tears flowed like the ocean as I walked on, sensing his hand in my hand, and imagining his sandals swinging from his other hand.

One of the most difficult things a widow has to deal with is what to do with the wedding ring (and the cell phone!). It's a heart wrenching decision for many. For me, it wasn't too difficult because I only ever wore my ring when I traveled, and I never left home without it on my ring finger. After Dave died, it was almost weird for me to put it on, and it was only an issue when I was off for a work trip, and I had to decide what to do, and then it became emotional. After a while, I stopped wearing it altogether. Widows and widowers see this issue differently. Some widows I have talked to continue to wear it on the right hand for many years, and some choose to have it made into another piece of jewelry. Dave bought me lots of fine jewelry over the years which I rarely wore, so I didn't want another piece. Widowers, many times, never wore it in the first place, so it wasn't a hard decision. As far as the cell phone, I kept it charged, and once every couple of days, I'd call it just to hear his voice; apparently this is not uncommon either!

One night after coming home from Cyndy Fitz's house right around the corner, I just started uncontrollably sobbing. I missed Dave, his larger-than-life presence, his love of me and of life, good wine, and good scotch! I missed him in my life. I missed hearing every day "Good Morning Beautiful!" Every day. And he really meant it. Don't get me wrong, there were challenges in our life as there are in every life together. But the underlying foundation of our relationship was true love, soulmate, fellow adventurer, fellow traveler, and just having a good time doing life together. A few times when I was feeling particularly lonely, I'd slip on his leather jacket, light a candle, and close my eyes to feel his presence.

When I first met Dave, we talked till three in the morning every night. We never stopped talking in thirty years. I still was able to make him laugh, and he loved to make me laugh! There was always something fresh, something new, and something different to talk and laugh about. I tell people that's one secret of a long marriage, keep laughing.

Dave always did the shopping at Costco; he was there at least every other week. I used to joke with him that we were only two people, and did he really need to super-size everything, especially Ketchup? After Dave died, I wanted to eliminate Costco from my life. It reminded me too much of Dave, his weekly trips, and most of all, I was now shopping for just one at this megastore. Toilet paper and paper towels were often on the Costco list, along with my large tin vats of Virginia peanuts (which I have since stopped eating), his big jar of mixed nuts, and huge boxes of granola bars (which I also stopped eating).

The challenge after he died became finding a new brand of toilet paper other than the leading Kirkland brand from Costco (according to Consumer Reports). I ran out of toilet paper, did my research, and found the leading selling toilet paper brand. I forget what brand it was, but it was supposedly sold at Walmart. So, there I was roaming the aisles looking for this brand on a Tuesday morning. I was still working at the time, and my manager Keith just happened to call me. I had to answer the phone. At that moment the "blue light special" announcement came on, very loudly, and I was busted. I had to explain what the heck I was doing in Walmart! It turned out he too had a toilet paper shopping experience and we both had a good laugh.

The stupid human tricks caused by the widow fog (like shaving only one leg and losing something every day) has settled down, thankfully. I believe the widow fog has lifted for good, and hopefully I'll never drive away again with the gas pump still attached to the car. Remember, find some smart friends. You're going to need them.

Losing a spouse, the love of your life, after spending half of your years on earth with him, changes every single thing. Nothing is the same, from waking up, to the morning rituals, cooking and sharing meals, the weekends, the evenings. The first year was spent mostly numb and in shock. Going through the motions of life, staggering around wondering what the hell just happened. Broken heart syndrome is real. It even has a name. Stress-induced cardiomyopathy.

So what does this loss of a spouse do to your stress level? If you're a caregiver, like me, you stop cooking and eating in front of your husband when he can't eat himself. I did manage to lose ten pounds, which was much needed but the wrong way to lose it (and I knew it wouldn't stay off, and it didn't). I knew I was overweight, but it never really bothered me, because I felt good, I was strong, Dave loved me just as I was, I worked out regularly, and tried to eat healthy.

Why is it that the loss of a spouse is the number one issue on the stress scale? And where exactly did the stress scale come from? Is it like the food pyramid that we've all believed our whole lives?

Everybody deals with the loss of a spouse differently. My fellow widow friends all shared stories about their loss. The reactions ranged from shaking fists at the sky even after thirty years, and screaming out loud to no one in particular "I could use some help down here!" One friend would put on country music and cry her eyes out. For me, the loss of affection, hugs, kisses, conversation, sleeping with someone in the buff, is the hardest thing. And do you really need to wait a year before you figure that out?

Many of the widows I met shared stories about how they were coping. The difference between men and women was striking.

For example, on the subject of dating, women often took years (if ever!) after their spouse passed away to even entertain the thoughts of seeing someone else. For widowers it was an average of six months, if that, before they were ready to be with someone else. One widower I spoke with said, "I just want someone to bring me an aspirin in the middle of the night." A lot of men are really babies when they get sick in the first place (I know Dave sure was). Another widower I know fell into the arms of a co-worker, and within three months, he was married again! I believe women are more scared and cautious before they even think about dating. Women tend to pick a new security system first, where men tend to pick a new spouse.

Have you heard this statement? *"You've got to get through one whole year!"* I always wondered what everyone meant when they said, "Don't make any decisions for a year!" Why a year? Would I magically wake up after one year and, POOF, be smart again? Would the widow fog lift? Would I be thin and desirable again? (The answer to all those questions was a resounding YES after a year!) Would I be thirty years old again? That I'm still working on. Not making a major decision for a year makes sense to me now, after experiencing all of the firsts and lasts of everything for myself the first year.

Debbie and Linda, both widows and good friends of mine, explained the one-year rule to me on Daytona Beach where we spent a week together. It's not just the first of everything—it's the lasts too, that get you. They were right. Our anniversary date, September 10, slammed me to the ground for two days. Made me retreat into my special place, all curled up and crying on the walk-in closet floor. Until you go through the firsts and lasts of everything, it's hard to know how it's going to hit you.

The last things we did together, experienced together, lived, and made memories from together, all hurt in different ways. "Have I told you today that I loved you?" The first day I didn't hear those words was very painful; there was a hole in my life and my heart where those words used to lift me up every day and make me smile.

For thirty years, Dave and I read the newspaper together. Heck, I grew up reading the newspaper even before my life with Dave. That habit came from Mom and Dad. When we lived in Canada, Dave would only read the sports section. After a while, he'd start reading every single section, front to back, leaving the comics and puzzles until the end, a reward.

Dave's last birthday was EPIC!! January 21 was his birthday, and Dave really loved a party. I surprised him for his 40th, 50th, and 60th birthdays, and there was no way I wasn't going to surprise him for this birthday, his last. As we got nearer to the date, a couple of people expressed discomfort with why I was doing this, knowing it was going to be Dave's last birthday, but they didn't know the history. So, one night, it got me thinking, maybe this was wrong after all. I got really upset, pacing all around the house. Dave sensed there was something terribly wrong. We had a strong connection and a sense of ESP together. (I never knew if he was reading my mind or if I was reading his, but it was uncanny.) He said to me, "Honey, what's up?" And I broke down, sobbing, and told him about the surprise party. I said, "Are you okay with this?" He wrapped me in his arms, calmed me down, and said, "It's okay, I love it. Go ahead."

I had three weeks to pull this event off, and of course a rare snowstorm happened in South Carolina which took a few days off the planning. The city of Charleston literally shut down for five days. As the short time went on, Dave knew there was going to be a party, but he had no idea how many or who was going to show up! Each night we sat on the front porch and night after night Dave asked me who was coming. I said, "We're up to forty." Then I'd say fifty and maybe sixty, adding as the event got closer. He was still feeling quite well, weak and losing weight like crazy because he couldn't eat much, but still positive and calm.

I had a lot of surprises up my sleeve! The party was on a Saturday night, and starting on Thursday night, each time the doorbell rang, I made Dave answer it, and I was ready with the camera rolling. I staged every arrival, the timing, and the lines they were going to tell Dave. Our incredible neighbors opened up their homes to house all of the out-of-town arrivals.

On Friday, the surprise visitors began with Jim and Dawn Jessen. We met them on our honeymoon thirty years before and although we kept in touch via Facebook, we hadn't seen them in years. The doorbell rang, Jim and Dawn, with drinks in hand, showed up and said, "Hey, we heard there was a party here!" And Dave said, "Well, nobody told me!" It became obvious Dave didn't know who they were, and when Dawn said, "You don't know who we are, do you?" Dave admitted it, and when she told him, he said his usual, "Jesus Christ, are you kidding me?!" and gave them both great big bear hugs.

There is a funny and beautiful story about Jim and Dawn and us going to a hockey tournament in Chatham, Ontario. They joined us from Detroit. Dawn was pregnant at the time with her beautiful daughter. Her doctor said she could only have one glass of wine. So we bought her a huge glass that would hold an entire bottle. We gave it to her and said, "Here's your one glass!" When they arrived for

Dave's birthday party, they brought this huge wine glass back which had just recently surfaced at their house. They had it etched: "Dave and Marie, Jim and Dawn, Forever Friends 1988." This special gift brought tears to our eyes after almost thirty years had passed.

The next arrival was my nephew Greg who Dave adored, and I know it was mutual. The doorbell rang and Dave answered it with Greg's nickname saying, "Crash!! What are you doing here?!" Everybody had a line, and Greg said, "Hey, I heard you needed help with your attic!" With tears in his eyes and his voice cracking, Dave introduced Greg to the growing crowd saying, "Everybody, this is Crash." Nephew Andrew rang the doorbell next, and of course Dave's comment was, "Oh, Jesus Christ!" giving him a big hug with the tears flowing again. It was Andrew who was one of my excuses for not having dinner with Dave back in 1987, he was born on our first date in Rochester. Peter and Maryann from Phoenix, Arizona, showed up next. They told Dave they were in the neighborhood and wouldn't have missed the party for the world! My sister arrived and that was a big surprise for me! The last planned arrival that evening was my dearest and oldest friend Anne from Campbell River, BC, who took four flights and all day to arrive. She rang the doorbell and said, "What's a girl gotta do to get a drink around here?" Well, Anne got the biggest and longest hug of the night!

The surprises continued the next day. Bob and Sue arrived on Saturday from Canada and so did Larry Wickens. These were Dave's oldest friends from their teenage years as Rover Scouts in Canada. Our old neighbors Kim and Mark were the last surprises and were standing in the kitchen as Dave came out after getting ready for the party.

Off we went to the birthday party at the club with almost 120 people having arrived for an epic party of dancing to an awesome DJ, eating ribeye steak dinner, and enjoying having lots of fun. The last Dave knew there were only forty–fifty people coming. The club where we lived, along with my wonderful friends, went all out to help me pull this off. We turned the corner and walked into the decorated pavilion. The look on his face was priceless, he was surprised, in tears, and left speechless at all the people who came out to help him celebrate his last birthday. The song for our entrance was the Beatles "They say it's your Birthday," and whenever I hear that song I smile.

Dave knew it was his last, and it was as if he wanted to set the example for me to continue to celebrate and embrace every precious minute of life.

The memories made that night helped us both get through the last months together. I took each of the videos made from each surprise arrival and made an iMovie that I treasure.

One of the last items on Dave's bucket list that he told me about while we were in Orlando was his desire to take flying lessons. I made that happen. This was about two months prior to his death, and he was still moving about just fine, and still feeling pretty good. My birthday gift to him was a private flying lesson at the Summerville airport. I kept it a surprise and he didn't know where we were going as I drove to the airport. The morning of the lesson we drove to the airport and met our pilot. Boy, was he surprised and beamed just like a little kid! He didn't even take pictures because he was so into the flight experience. I was so glad to make this finally happen for you, Dave.

Our friend Deb surprised Dave with another special gift which I managed to keep a surprise, just like the flying lesson. Dave was a sports fan, especially baseball. We talked about going to a college game for years but never made it. The surprise was a University of South Carolina Gamecocks baseball game in Columbia, South Carolina. Deb was a season ticket holder and we sat in the famous Coach Tanner's suite. I'll never forget Coach Tanner walking into the suite, saying hello, and Dave standing up with Coach Tanner saying hello back. The coach said, "It's okay, you don't have to stand." Dave said, "I'm in the presence of baseball royalty, and I will most certainly stand up!" He had a knack for remembering sports statistics like nobody else, and he knew the Coach's storied history.

Thinking back on our life together, the lesson for me was your bucket list should never be postponed. You never know how much time you might have left on this earth to experience the chance to make memories. I looked back and realized there was nothing left on the bucket list that we hadn't done, at least that I knew of, except maybe golfing in Scotland.

My last birthday at the club was in March, the month before he died. We were supposed to go up for dinner, but we headed up for dessert instead. By that point, Dave wasn't interested in food, and I didn't like to eat in front of him, feeling it was too cruel. I didn't even want to go, but I'm so glad I did. I was surprised with wonderful birthday cards, flowers, and laughs, and surrounded by good friends. Our friend Bill made a birthday cake which said "Happy Brithday," not catching the typo!

Earlier that same night, Dave was sitting on the front porch in tears because he couldn't get out to buy me a card for the first time ever in our life together. He couldn't drive anymore, so he didn't get to a store. Broke my heart into little pieces! Worse though, he was gone seventeen days later.

The last real dinner Dave ate was at one of our favorite restaurants in Charleston called Coast with three other couples. It was on March 17, St. Patty's Day, where we went after seeing the play *Avenue Q, The Musical*. He was so excited to eat three whole scallops! The night before was at Dennis and Marilyn's and he ate well there too. But the scallops were the last dinner. It's funny how the little details are the ones we remember most strongly.

There were a lot of lasts. Your last scotch was with Bill Gardiner sitting in the sunroom. The last time you woke up and said, "Good morning beautiful!" The last time you woke up and said you felt terrific which you did every morning. The last time you put your hand on my hip, your favorite spot, where you'd rest it every night.

After Dave died, I had so many decisions to make, all by myself, and in a short timeframe.

Cars and trucks were the next thing to deal with after Dave died. I felt like I was flying solo by the seat of my pants, making stuff up as I moved through each and every day. There wasn't anyone to bounce decisions by, and the reality that I was alone became a heavy weight to bear. My car was fourteen years old, and I sold it with only 36,500 miles on it. How could the miles be so low? Because Dave drove around every day doing EVERY SINGLE THING—grocery shopping, shuttling me back and forth to the airport for my work travels, car maintenance, golf days, or returning stuff for me to stores using his truck. My friend Deb called me a catch and release shopper. I would find something to buy, bring it home, try it on again, and realize I had to release it back into the shopping universe.

Was there a moment I felt it was time to march forward and embrace life again? It may have been when I decided to sell Dave's beloved 1967 Corvette Stingray convertible which he restored from the ground up. I had to; with the racing clutch, it took two legs to push the clutch in, you needed arm power to shift (not that I didn't have the strength!), and the car had to be driven and not just constantly parked. I knew I couldn't sit around and let that beautiful classic collect dust, a reason to make sure it went to a good place where it would be driven. With no trunk, black leather seats, and no A/C, it wasn't even practical in the south. We didn't really take it anywhere except to the beach once a year when we moved from the north to the south. Neighbor Eason and his son Chandler helped me create a couple of videos to help sell the car.

When it left the garage for the last time, it stopped my heart, I couldn't breathe, and the tears flowed down my cheeks. This vehicle had been a part of my life too for thirty years. One time, driving it home down Airport Road from Collingwood to Mississauga, a rainstorm started, and of course the top was down. These two older ladies drove up beside us and both were grinning with thumbs up because we were smiling, soaked, and it just didn't matter! We had many memories in that turquoise blue Corvette.

My first New Year's Eve alone was in Sarasota for a black-tie gala. I didn't have a date, and I didn't want one. I felt it was time to get dressed up and go to a party even though I had nothing to celebrate. We spent hours getting ready into our gowns, and we arrived fashionably late.

Right before midnight, I snuck out to the front yard to be alone and not have to kiss anyone. Staring up at the sky, I saw Orion, our favorite constellation, and it was bittersweet. Two of my friends came looking for me and found me in tears, but they both understood why, being widows themselves. To tell you the truth, the best part of that night was actually getting ready. Hair, makeup, and girlfriends—what a great combination.

As if the life changes that come with losing your spouse aren't enough, I also needed an oil change. I remember looking up at the little decal the service station put on the windshield and realized— Holy Crud—I needed an oil change, like four months ago! That was a shocker. I screamed with my fists raised to the sky and yelled, "THIS IS NOT MY JOB!"

It took me a while after Dave died to put the music back on again. One day I asked Siri to play me some music and I was shocked at the choices made. The songs she chose were not even on any of my playlists and took my breath away. The first one was Jive Aces "Bring Me Sunshine." Dave made everyone we knew watch the YouTube video of this song, whether they wanted to or not. And if you didn't smile by the end of this song, there was something wrong. The second one was from Sade, another longtime favorite of ours. Sade was a romantic singer, and Dave was a romantic soul. Next up was a Blues Brothers song, a movie we've seen at LEAST fifty times. It was followed by another longtime favorite by Louis Prima, an artist Dave adored. His favorite song from Louis had the lyrics "I eat antipasta twice just because you are so nice!" Finally, the next song came on with the lyrics "Chitlin and grits washed down with a swallow of scotch!" Dave's favorite drink of all time was scotch with three ice cubes, no more, no less. Again, these were not songs in my playlist.

They were songs Siri pulled out of the air, or maybe it was Dave living on in spirit, at work to make me smile.

I was still working from home as much as I could with my diminished brain power. I told my boss Keith I was ready to slowly ease back into travel after a few months passed, thinking it would be a good distraction. I had a great job which I loved as an HR and payroll sales consultant. This meant I got to travel around, find out customer pains and issues, then tailor and deliver product demonstrations sometimes in two or three cities a week. I used to say it's a great gig for frustrated actresses because each demo was a performance, sometimes even on stage if it was a large group.

My first work trip I had was to Los Angeles for a customer demo. I had fond memories of California and the many places visited for work and for pleasure. Flying was weird all of a sudden, no one to text or call that you arrived, no one to tell you "I love you" and "Fly safe," and no one to pick me up at the airport on the return home. Coming home to a dark empty house was not appealing either. I did make it to Santa Monica beach on that trip, and walked it, sensing Dave by my side holding my hand. The next day, I had a breakdown in the airport coming home. It was a costly breakdown that led me to spend another $900 out of my pocket to buy a ticket home because I messed up the reservation badly. Coming home made me very sad, especially late at night.

I started buying one-way tickets because there was no reason to come home anymore. I didn't even feel like it was my "home" anymore. I would extend my trips for sometimes weeks at a time; I had no reason to come home to an empty house. I craved conversation. I craved our social life. Singing at the top of our lungs with friends. Dancing outside under the pavilion at our favorite club. Dancing in the kitchen. Dancing period. I missed all those things you do with your partner in life for a long, long time.

One trip, I bought a one-way ticket to Toronto for work, then to Boise, Idaho, for a customer demonstration, then flew up to see my friend Anne in Vancouver for one night. The next day we took Beaver Air over to Vancouver Island and had a lovely couple of days hiking the trails near her house on the ocean. It was a good distraction being away and being with my best friend Anne, but it didn't make coming home after two weeks any easier.

Bob and Kathy Richards invited me to join them and another couple up at the club for Mother's Day brunch which we always enjoyed together. The table was set for six, but there were only five of us. It takes my breath away every time the realization hits that you're single now, no longer part of a couple. I did a double take at the empty seat, thinking to myself—*where's Dave?* I was expecting you to be by my side, but you weren't. Getting used to flying solo was not easy at all.

Sundays are the worst day of the week for me since he died on a Sunday morning. Saturdays are the second worst. Our weekends were special—friends, cooking, dancing, golfing, entertaining, and I missed that the most. I actually started inviting girl friends over for dinner just to get back to cooking, which always made my soul happy. This was a simple step I took which helped bring back some joy into my life. One night, the girls came over and we had a "BYOM" party which stood for Bring Your Own Meat. We sat and grilled out on the back deck and had a wonderful evening sipping wine, cooking, chatting, and eating.

Dave was like a little kid on holidays. He loved the Anniversary bunny, birthday bunny, Christmas bunny, Easter bunny, cards and flowers and chocolate! In fact, he'd buy me flowers for Valentine's Day along with a box of chocolates, and inevitably it would be *his* favorite chocolates. I do miss his love of the holidays, both big and small. The first year of holidays spent without him made me miss him sorely. The Easter bunny and Santa were not real, but Dave was, and he was gone.

One of the first things I did at the house was install a security system. Even though for thirty years, if there was a strange noise, I was the brave one to get up and check. After Dave died, I felt unprotected and scared. I was scared of burglars, animals, strange men, and mischievous teenagers. The security system gave me peace of mind being home alone. There were cameras all around the perimeter and a monitor which I could check at any time, and I checked it a lot. It never did diminish my fear of being alone though.

Christmas Eve 2018 was my first Christmas Eve alone. This went along with another first which wasn't pleasant either, in fact it was downright scary. It was a house emergency with no man around. It came very close to burning the house down. This just happens to be my biggest fear in life. The night before, I smelled something burning, like plastic. I thought it was because I hadn't changed the air filters, ever. I woke up Christmas Eve morning and realized the heat wasn't on. Called my smart friend Linda (remember, everybody needs to surround themselves with smart friends) and I said, "Hey, what do you think could be wrong?"

She said, "I bet you it's the battery." So, she came over, and we tried to wrestle the thermostat off the wall, which wasn't easy. But we did manage it, and found the battery inside the unit. Linda just happened to have one in her drawer that was the right size. We replaced the battery but that didn't make it work. Then we got neighbors John and Mike to come over and look at it, and they said you need a new thermostat! So off to Home Depot I go on Christmas Eve morning and buy myself a thermostat. Thank goodness for the workers there who were very helpful. I brought the thermostat home, got the old one off, and the guys figured out how to rewire it. A couple of hours later and a little splash of paint to cover up the holes, and lo and behold, it still didn't work, no heat yet. I was very lucky to find an A/C local guy who came over, on Christmas Eve especially. He found the heater unit up in the attic totally melted down and burned to pieces; that was the smell coming out of the heater I noticed the night before. This totally freaked me out, but the wonderful A/C technician did get the heat back on for which I was thankful.

My friend Linda had planned three days and nights of events at her house for the holidays, right across the golf course from my house. I was going to Linda's that day and after the guys left, I proceeded to have a meltdown. How could this be happening to me? I cried out to the empty house. After so many years of having Dave the fireman around fixing everything, this incident was especially painful. It left me feeling helpless. My life had burned down around me and now the house almost did too.

At that exact moment, dear Cindy just happened to come over for a visit, gave me a big hug, with a lot of tears spilled, and took charge, calmed me down, and helped me get ready for my first Christmas Eve alone. I had a platter of food I was taking over to Linda's and a side dish, and she just finished it all for me. The power of friends—they always come through and sense when you need it the most.

There are only two certainties in life: death and taxes. That year I had both! The first-time doing taxes alone, I felt just like my friend Cyndy when she'd shake her fists at the sky at her late husband and yell at him. (He coincidentally died of the same cancer as Dave but at the very young age of thirty-four years.) I did the same as she did, and yelled out, "I could use a little help down here!" This was another thing that was totally Dave's job; he did the taxes every year. Taxes for us were complicated because they included two countries—US and Canada. They never got filed until late that first year. I'm working very hard to make sure all the following years are filed on time.

Some firsts included my first Valentine's alone for which I cooked dinner for my girlfriends. We all were single and all widowed. We got through the most romantic night of the year together, and I was grateful for that. The first Thanksgiving alone, I flew to Phoenix to meet up with my friends—Anne, Mark and Laura, and Peter and Maryann. It was the first time I saw them since Dave died. This was a special group of friends who were by my side the entire journey.

My first work trip to New York City alone was hard; it was one of our favorite places and we were there at least twice a year. I was there for a team meeting and went two days early to get the emotions out of my system. I visited our timeshare on West 57th, walked the streets of Manhattan, went to our favorite Italian restaurant, and managed to get the last ticket in the house to Sunday's *Hamilton* show two nights before departing. When Dave and I were there on a couple of our trips, we tried to get tickets but didn't because of the cost. I swear Dave was looking over my shoulder when I got this ticket—Row F, seat 110—at the exact center of the theater. As an added bonus, I was surrounded by short people. It was the best show I've ever seen in my life. Dave would've loved every song and every minute.

I bought a new grill, because for some reason, every grill we ever owned had a malfunctioned starter! Dave, like most men, was the griller in the house. The first time I was grilling steaks for Linda and me on the new grill, there was a bright red cardinal who landed in the tree who stayed there the whole time. I looked up and said, "I know, I know, Dave! Four minutes a side. I got this!"

Sept 10, 2018, would have been our 30th anniversary, and this is what I wrote in my journal:

> *Today I cry tears of happiness to have joined hands in marriage thirty years ago today to the man who told me over and over through the years "If you wanted easy, you could have married anyone!!" Spent half my life having one "Dave and Marie Adventure" after another. Lots of laughs, lots of love.*
>
> *Today I cry tears of sadness, because you are no longer physically here with me, Dave. I loved you with all my heart and soul. Your energy and presence are still here with me.*
>
> *Today I cry tears of gratitude to know that over the past thirty years, we never only celebrated on one special day, we celebrated the whole year, like our dear friends Marv and Donna. What that means is we started celebrating our 30th year together LAST September every chance we had for the entire year.*

The last of the firsts and lasts came from April 15, 2019, and this is what I wrote:

And then there was one. One night left on this earth – and we didn't know it.

Last night I sat on the front porch in your rocking chair and relived every minute of that day and night. The visits and calls from everyone from morning till night was as if the universe rallied all to say goodbye. But we didn't know it was the last. Maryann and Peter helped me get you to bed, propped your legs up on pillows. You thought the swelling in your leg and hip was a blood clot, so all night long almost unconsciously you did your foot pumps, just like they taught you in rehab for your two knees and hip replacements. You were so sick and restless that night I crept out of bed and watched over you from the bedroom chair in the corner. In one of your lucid moments, you woke up and patted my side of the bed which you did a million times during our thirty years. It was about 2:00 a.m. and said, "Honey, I had to feel my pulse to make sure I wasn't dead, because you weren't there!" I came back to bed in silent tears and held you close in my arms until 6:00 a.m. when I went and woke up Maryann to come help. I put on Soundscapes on the music channel thinking it might soothe you. I can't listen to this channel to this day!

Dave, all you wanted to do was get to the front porch one more time that morning, but we couldn't get you out there. You took your last breath peacefully in my arms at 8:32. I'll never ever forget that precious moment; it's the most powerful and memorable moment of my life which I'll cherish forever. I sat on the front porch for you last night and then again in the morning.

And then there was one. One last first to go through this year, the first anniversary of your leaving this earth. I love you,

Dave Scott—always did from our first date on May 2, 1987, and I always will.

February happened to be our last vacation together, a cruise out of Fort Lauderdale. Almost exactly a year after that, I'm on my way to Egypt for my first solo adventure. I joined dear friends Mark and Laura who were with us on Dave's last cruise as well as the last three years of Flower Power cruises. We met them on a Baltic capitals cruise where we spent each night at the piano bar singing and dancing. The trip was amazing. We flew out of JFK and into Cairo for three nights, cruised the Nile for three nights, and spent three nights in Luxor. I felt like I was seeing Egypt through two sets of eyes, and I really believe Dave was by my side the whole trip. I wear a small necklace with some of Dave's ashes in it—it's pretty special. One time going through security, I had a full-frontal pat down and the agent said, "IS THIS A MICROPHONE!" I swear I could hear Dave laughing, and saying, "Yes dear, speak louder into the microphone!" I calmly said, "No, it's just a necklace." I knew that it was frowned upon to travel with ashes, so I didn't dare say it was a piece of my husband.

It reminds me of all the memories we made around the world. I learned how important memories are when you lose someone close; it's all you have left. I will always continue to make memories the rest of my life; they're so important and mean so much. So thankful for our memories captured in thousands and thousands of pictures.

Dave always said to leave a little sand from the beach in your shoes, that way you know you'll be back, and I do at every beach I visit.

365 days and nights was gone in the blink of an eye. Yes, I do believe it is better to have loved and lost than never have loved before.

Life as a widow sucks. It's a life of a lot of firsts and lasts. Some actually experience worse grief in their second year, which I didn't know how to process and didn't want to, as the first year was bad enough. But there are no rules and no timetable; each person grieves differently.

You've got to get through one whole year! I did, they were right, and it's going to be alright. I felt this in my bones and my heart and my soul. What came next in my life was an unexpected transformation.

CHAPTER 6

A New Marie, High on Organic Vegetables

"Let food be thy medicine and medicine be thy food."
—Hippocrates

Was there really a link between food and medicine? Could I have helped Dave?

Dave's cancer diagnosis led me down the path of learning more about the concept of "Food as Medicine." In my desperate attempt to help Dave, the seed about food as medicine was planted in my mind, and I started reading. We were desperate for any hope at all. We all have heard and read stories of miraculous recoveries from stage four cancer, and one I knew was actually a co-worker. He turned to juicing and documented his journey to overcome this terrible disease.

The biggest and scariest thing I learned back then was the link between sugar, processed foods which have high sugar content, and cancer cell growth.

Sugar feeds cancer. Period.

After my mom died, I also sought out to learn more about the link between food and Alzheimer's. This made me doubly interested in learning more about nutrition. Studies have shown the link between aluminum and Alzheimer's. Maybe the old aluminum pots with tomato sauce cooking in them all day long contributed to Mom's diagnosis.

Oracle, my long-time employer, started a "Healthy Weight Challenge" years ago, and I jumped in with both feet (my very heavy feet). I weighed in at 161 pounds which I had been carting and carrying around with me for a very long time. As the years went by, thirty pounds crept on, and I just figured it was due to the normal aging process.

This weight challenge, about seven years before Dave died, started me out on working with a trainer, and I continue to do this. It's like a date and I never miss going. It's my motivation to get there, and I recommend it to anyone wanting to start some kind of routine by having an accountability partner like a trainer. I'd occasionally also work out as a team with my friend Deb, who had embarked on a "Whole30" diet. I remember her saying she forgot how good a real strawberry or blueberry tasted until she went organic. After many years of working out with a trainer, I didn't lose a pound, my weight stayed the same, but I did start thinking more about food.

My trainer at the YMCA talked to me a lot about nutrition, and what you put in your mouth was just as important as working out and exercising. She introduced me to the world of Paleo and ancestral eating. While Dave and I had followed a low carb Atkins food plan for many years, we were still eating processed food, a lot of bacon, gluten free pasta, gluten free breads, sweets (when dining out), and not enough raw foods.

Tearing my rotator cuff, a year before Dave was diagnosed with cancer, began my path to move away from traditional medicine and more toward functional medicine. This, unknowingly, became the turning point for my health transformation, including weight loss, fitness awareness, and general well-being. The last regular doctor's visit I had was a year earlier, and solely focused on two things during our allotted fifteen minutes, cholesterol and blood pressure.

The big fall happened one late night before Dave and I were scheduled to depart to Honolulu early the next morning for a week-long work trip. We tacked on a couple days of vacation before and after this work trip because we both loved Hawaii. I had just returned earlier that day from a work trip to Denver, and I was so proud of myself for getting unpacked, and then repacked for the Hawaii trip.

This moment is etched on my brain. I got all our bags downstairs for an early morning departure. I reached around Dave to turn on the hall light to go upstairs to bed and tripped over a suitcase, falling hard on the hall floor, and jamming my right shoulder. I lay there crying and screaming in agony knowing I did something bad, and Dave's fire training immediately took over. He calmed me down, assessed that nothing was broken, and said to me through his tears, "What do you want to do?" and I said, "Well, let's go." The next morning, we headed to Honolulu on a ten-hour flight with my arm propped up between us on blankets. I couldn't lift it at all. He didn't take his eyes off me for the entire trip. The next day, I found a clinic in Honolulu where the doctor took an X-ray and confirmed Dave's diagnosis that it was not broken. When I got back home, an MRI confirmed a 75% tear in the rotator cuff, a tear in the bicep, and that my A/C joint had rheumatoid arthritis as well. I was told at the time that a torn rotator cuff that bad could not be healed, 50% maybe, but not 75% like mine.

When we returned home, I began physical therapy at two different places with no measurable gain in range of motion. I still couldn't lift my arm up to my shoulder, and certainly couldn't golf or work out, let alone wash my own hair. After months of hearing about an amazing Chiropractor, Dr. Jeremiah Jimerson, recommended by my trainer at the YMCA and also through my friends in the neighborhood, I made an appointment. Using A.R.T. (Active Release Therapy), Dr.

Jimerson totally and completely rehabbed my shoulder to better than ever before. His therapy really hurt, and it did take about six months, but it was worth every minute of pain. He also taught me so much more, like how to be "bulletproof," so if I fell again, I'd be more prepared to not get injured again. He taught me about proper form for doing deadlifts, many different stretches, and most importantly he taught me how to belly breathe. I have so much gratitude for Dr. Jimerson in my life, and glad I made that first appointment. I call him "Magic Man" and he's helped with so many other things as well, like my golfer's elbow, weak hip flexors, my knees, and back. I was determined to find another path to health.

After Dave died, I continued my work with Dr. Jimerson. He introduced me to an Osteopath who was working at his practice, and it was my first real encounter with the world of functional medicine. I learned functional medicine stressed getting to the root cause of health issues, like my pre-diabetes linked to a diet high in carbs (not so much sugar which I didn't eat anyway).

Everyone knows the basics of health, like an apple a day keeps the doctor away and don't eat too many potato chips (my weakness). I did not really understand the power of the human body to heal itself. How's this for a trivia answer: did you know the human species is the only one that doesn't self-regulate its weight? Think about it, have you ever seen an obese tiger or overweight zebra in the wild?

It was also the first time ever in my life someone asked not only about me and my health history, but also my family's health history. This was eye-opening. I realized all the autoimmune diseases running rampant in my family could happen to me too, especially after being misdiagnosed with Autoimmune Hepatitis years before. Sister Jean had Celiac, sister Kathy had Graves, brother Mike had Hypothyroidism, brother George died of ALS (aka Lou Gehrig's disease)—all autoimmune diseases. Continuing with the family health history, Mom was a diabetic, had multiple strokes, and several heart attacks when she was in her '60s. She spent the rest of her life on about fifteen medications a day. Dad had one heart attack, fixed it with a stent, took his prescriptions for exactly one month, and stopped!

The Osteopath left the practice, and for months I'd keep asking Dr. Jimerson how I was going to find another natural doctor. Right after one of our visits for my shoulder, he was standing at his laptop recapping his notes, and just happened to mention almost under his breath "Living Proof Institute" (LPI) founded by Sachin Patel.

Little could I have imagined what was about to happen!

I went home, googled LPI, and the next week I had an introductory call. I was quite worried I wasn't going to be accepted into the program, but I think they sensed I was in the "action" stage of change and accepted me into their "Essentials Program." I flew to Toronto to meet Dr. Navaz Habib the next week, and also had a call with a health coach, to talk about diet and nutrition. Because of the autoimmune issues I had and the family history, I was put on the Paleo AIP (autoimmune protocol) food plan which I still follow. The weight (thirty pounds) melted away after six short weeks, and it's stayed off to this day. No one can believe my birth age; I am fit, healthy, and most importantly, my daily energy level is through the roof!

When I got involved with the Living Proof Institute, I also started studying self-care like meditation, massage, stress reduction, and mindfulness. My health transformation began by healing from the inside. Finding the Living Proof Institute opened my eyes to the impact of grief on my mental and physical states. I was better able to deal with Dave's loss in many ways with many different tools I could practice.

Dr. Habib also ordered a series of tests when we began working together, such as the Organic Acids Test, the Dutch Test, Glyphosate, and the GI Map. Some of the results uncovered included chronic stress, crashing adrenals, high levels of Glyphosate (hello good old Round-up!), hormones out of whack, and a couple of nasty bugs. He had a saying, "Don't worry. Anything we can measure, we can fix!" This we did over the next six months. All of the stress from caregiving for Dave through his surgeries, many ER visits, and his final journey, I'm sure, contributed to my chronic stress diagnosis. When the testing I went through with the Living Proof Institute uncovered this, among other issues, I was told "Stress is the most serious issue, AND you need to do something about this NOW before you crash and burn." So I took up meditation as one way to help calm down. It was very beneficial to my healing in so many other ways as well. It taught me how to just pause and breathe for a moment or two throughout the day.

Through a variety of life changes, I have managed to reverse many of the other autoimmune conditions my testing and diagnosis uncovered. Nutrition was the most significant change and created the greatest impact. I try to eat clean, organic, whole foods, grass fed beef, organic chicken, and wild caught seafood, especially salmon. You can always find a piece of salmon and a salad in most restaurants around the world!

If it wasn't for my two exceptional doctors, Dr. Jimerson in South Carolina, and Dr. Habib in Toronto, I'd be depressed and for sure on antidepressants (that's a first line of order for doctors to treat grief), still on blood pressure medications, on Metformin because I was pre-diabetic, unfit, overweight, taking phentermine for weight loss, cholesterol drugs (my magic "number" skyrocketed to 299), on estradiol for Hormone Replacement Therapy, and I'm sure I'd be drinking too much. Today I take nothing but a few supplements. Not even Advil which I used to call "Golfer's Aid" to get me through a round of golf. I used to live on Imodium for diarrhea, especially when I was on the road, and haven't needed that since. It's no longer on my Costco shopping list and out of every cupboard and purse.

I was on my way to good health, a place I thought I was already at!

People are intrigued and some are inspired by my lifestyle changes, my health transformation, and my body transformation. I went from a size XL shirt (which NO ONE could believe—I hid it well) to a small, and pants from a size fourteen to a six. When I first got down to a size ten, I was so happy, especially because it was the first time in twenty years I had been that weight. I thought, this is great! And I went shopping. Then, I got down to a size eight and went shopping again. Next size down was to a size six where I remain to this day. I'm satisfied here at this weight, not to mention I don't want to go shopping for another size! This is the weight I was when I met Dave back in 1986, and he'd absolutely love the transformation.

Maya Angelou said, "People forget what you said, and what you did, but they'll never forget how you made them feel." Dave made me feel beautiful and special every single day for thirty years. He had unconditional love for me; fat, skinny, long hair, short hair, makeup, no makeup—it didn't matter.

I couldn't save Dave, but now I had the tools to save myself. After deciding to embrace life again, and march forward with one foot in front of the other, Life Part Two for me next meant diving into finding my new purpose in life. My new clarity of purpose, and my driving force for everything I've done since Dave died, became this vision: "Help and inspire widows and widowers to live well, laugh more, and love again."

I was ready for a new mission, but had no clue what was around the corner.

CHAPTER 7

"7 Steps to Healing After Loss"

I hadn't even been through the firsts and lasts of life after Dave died before I was slammed to the floor again. That same year, I was hit by another battering ram of grief when I lost my mom, the beautiful Faye Bailey. Mother of eight, wife to my dad, George (he died eight years before), and grandmother and aunt to countless others. After these two life altering events, I was a real blast to be around.

Joyce Brothers, in her book *Widowed* (friend Cyndy Fitz told me to buy this and I'm glad I did) said, "A weeping widow is as popular as a case of the flu." Tears actually have a chemical which is the body's natural pain reliever, as ugly as it can be. Small consolation, I know.

Mom's death drove me even more to focus on self-care, eating right to feel good, and learning more about nutrition and the link to chronic diseases. Especially the ones running through my family like cancer, diabetes, and Alzheimer's.

The "7 Steps to Healing After Loss" became my mantra and desire to help others after Dave died, and these same steps helped me deal with the loss of my dear mom. Living alone without Dave made me come to realize I had to love myself first, and I did, by healing my mind, body, and spirit.

Today I still lie on the floor and stare at the ceiling, mostly to meditate, be grateful, and do yoga poses which all have been a part of my healing process.

Step 1: Leverage Food as Medicine

How did I get well? The short answer is through Functional Medicine. It will forever change the way I approach my health. Going through the agony of cancer with Dave, and the numerous doctors he had to see, made me realize there was something missing from traditional medicine. I wanted someone to help me figure out WHY he got cancer in the first place. This shifted my feeling about my healthcare and learning how traditional medicine was really "sick care." Here's a good description on what traditional medicine is, from a quote from an honest doctor who said, "If I put you on a pill, I could see you back every three months for the rest of your life. That's how we make money in medicine. But if I change your eating preferences and you get healthy, I may never see you again!" How true is that?

I got to thinking about my last regular doctor's appointment. It was back in 2016 before Dave died; and in the course of the usual allotted fifteen minutes of a "wellness" visit, the doctor focused on only two things, my cholesterol and blood pressure numbers. Not one question about my energy levels, what I was eating (they don't learn about that in medical school anyway!), or how I could correct these issues with lifestyle changes instead of pills. I left that day with two new prescriptions, one for blood pressure and another for cholesterol.

Trivia answer: Did you know cholesterol is the biggest selling class of pharma drugs of all time? It's taken by hundreds of millions of people around the world, but not me anymore!

Functional medicine has also given me a good foundation to help ensure my family legacy of longevity. (The only good thing about my crappy family health history is that longevity runs in the family!) I want to still be golfing at age ninety and shooting a good score with my full mental faculties still intact. I truly want to die young at an old age.

What is the description of Functional Medicine? It is true "health" care and not "sick" care. It stresses the prevention of chronic disease through finding the root cause of the symptoms and also stresses food as nutrition. Traditional healthcare is really "sick" care, there to give you a prescription for a symptom like a headache, prescription for high cholesterol, prescription for blood pressure, prescription for hormones. But it's not trying to find out WHY you have these symptoms. Before you know it, you're on multiple medications with no exit strategy whatsoever. That's what happened to me. That's what happened to my mother. She had diabetes among other things and took three to five different medications to control her blood sugar alone. And of course, none of her doctors spoke to each other, the heart doctor, the gut doctor, her primary care doctor, or her stroke doctors. That's the difference between traditional and functional medicine. You have a symptom? We have a pill for that! Name it (Diabetes). Tame it (three different pills). Blame it (oh, I have no energy, it's my diabetes!). Functional medicine gets to the root of the cause, and stresses nutrition as the first line of battle.

Losing Dave motivated me to take control of what I COULD control—my health.

I eat well every single day, cooking most meals at home, and always with leftovers for the next day's lunch. Even though I had always cooked and eaten well, I was eating the wrong things. I had been gluten free for years, but still eating gluten free stuff out of a box or a bag, still highly processed food and high in carbs. I learned how to read a food label and was appalled at how many ingredients in supposedly "healthy" foods you couldn't pronounce.

For me it became so simple—don't eat stuff out of a box.

I eat organic for a few reasons, the two biggest being the strict government standards for getting that USDA label (in the US), and the taste! If you've never had an organic strawberry or an organic blueberry, the taste is purer and sweeter. I remember my friend Deb who was on the "Whole 30" food plan saying, "I forgot how a blueberry tasted until I bought an organic pint."

Organic fruit and vegetables are grown without chemicals or synthetic pesticides, under strict guidelines about crop rotation, weed killers, and soil condition. The US Department of Agriculture, with their USDA label, certifies the food you are eating is truly organic, and not genetically modified to improve crop yield or prevent diseases of the crops. These pesticides are used widely with little to no care given to the side effects on the human body. A prime example is cancer-causing glyphosate, commonly sold in the US as "Roundup." It is banned in many countries, including most of Europe, except the US. When I was tested with extremely high levels of glyphosate, this became one of my biggest motivations to eat organic. I was horrified that I'd been eating such dangerous chemicals and had no idea what it could do to the human body.

In the beginning, I was totally overwhelmed with all the information I was learning about my poor eating habits. I'd spent my life believing I was "healthy." I needed some help. A great start was the EWG (Environmental Working Group) who publishes "The Dirty Dozen" and the "Clean 15" focusing on which products to always go organic with, and the Clean 15 which are lesser evils in terms of the pesticides used. For example, you should always splurge on organic strawberries, kale, and spinach. Products with the fewest pesticides include avocados, asparagus, and onions. You can find the full list on their website, EWG.org.

On the fitness front, for many years I was working out with a trainer twice a week. I walked the golf course every single weekend. I walked the neighborhood every other day, making sure I got my 10,000–15,000 steps in every single day. My best friend Anne gave me my first Fitbit back many years before, and I also used many varieties of pedometers, yet I never lost a pound. I was okay with that, and so was Dave, but of course he had unconditional love for me no matter what I weighed, no matter if my hair was short or long, and no matter if I wore makeup or not! We tried many diets, the usual suspects like Weight Watchers, Atkins, Gundry, and South Beach. Nothing worked.

It wasn't until I was introduced to Sachin Patel's Living Proof Institute (chapter 6), that my health transformation began. Yes, I was fit and strong because of golf, walking, and working out, but I had no idea how far away I was from being truly healthy. As I learned more and more, I was able to articulate the many ways to heal, and by embracing the "7 Steps to Healing," my own body, mind, and spirit began a radical transformation I never thought was possible.

Until you focus on your own health, it's very hard to overcome the tremendous grief a loss like this causes, both emotionally and physically.

For one thing, I could never shed the extra thirty pounds I was carrying no matter what I did or what diet I was trying. I started gaining this weight back in the mid '90s, and I attributed it to having quit smoking three times, so I was okay with that tradeoff. For a good twenty years, I weighed in at 161 pounds, and at five feet, three inches, that made me officially overweight.

As I changed my food preferences, my body shrunk dramatically (those thirty pounds melted away in the short time span of six weeks), and my friends asked me early on, what the heck do you eat? I wanted to show them the power of incredible, nutrient rich whole foods, so I just invited them over to my house for dinner instead. My love of cooking and entertaining helped me find joy by this simple act of having friends over for dinner. It also became a pivotal way to manage my grief; eating dinner with someone is a proven health booster, mentally and physically.

A big purchase I made for my kitchen was to invest in a whole kitchen full of colorful cast iron pots and pans. They make me smile when I cook and motivate me to be creative and inventive in the kitchen. I'll look at a pot and envision a roasted chicken in a dutch oven, or perhaps a cast iron seared ribeye. These help drive my creativity in picking and trying new recipes for my future cookbook. I still try to cook every night at home, just like I did with Dave. If you aren't cooking at home, it's hard to eat clean when you're dining out all the time. Too many temptations!

Just as important as what you eat, it's also how you eat. Sachin Patel, in one of his "30 Ways in 30 Days" video tips (www.30in30. org), advises "Chill, Chew and Cherish." The body has two states. The first is "rest and digest" and the second is "fight or flight." If you're not relaxed, you're not digesting your food properly. So no more snacking at the kitchen counter standing up, of which I was guilty as charged. (My mom always said, "Don't eat standing up, your ankles will get fat!") Chew your food almost to mush before you swallow because digestion begins in the mouth. Remember Gomer Pyle? Well, his grandma always said, "Chew Yer Food twelve times." Finally, cherish your food by giving thanks—for the meal in front of you, to the farmers who helped grow the food on your plate, to the stores that keep their shelves stocked. Sitting down to dinner and being present reminded me of Dave and how we remained present with each other in each and every moment at the end of his life.

As an added bonus, these three tips have helped to heal my gut and keep me regular!

The first suggestion made to me by my health coach was to clean out my pantry. I thought cleaning the pantry would be a slam dunk, easy peasy. Anything had to be easier than cleaning out Dave's closet. I always thought I ate healthy, but apparently not. I started reading labels on the boxes and bags stored on my pantry shelves, and I was astonished as to what I was putting in my body. Half the ingredients were unrecognizable. One of the first rules of reading a label is if you can't pronounce it, then you probably shouldn't eat it. The second rule is the fewer ingredients the better. At the same time, I was diagnosed with a gluten intolerance, I learned about alternative flours like Cassava and Almond flour and learned how to cook with avocado oil instead of olive oil. Avocado oil can be used to cook at a much higher temperature than olive oil. The smoke point is 480 degrees vs 350 for olive oil, and I never knew this important fact. This makes olive oil best for your salads and for low cooking, but not high heat cooking. Please don't tell Mom; we grew up with everything cooked in olive oil or lard. Oh yes, and who could forget the unnaturally colored margarines of my youth.

As I was learning to navigate a new life alone, I also learned I was shopping all wrong. Today, my shopping trips are spent mostly on the outside aisles, and always with a list! Most of the items in my cart are from the produce department, seafood, and the meat section. I try to stay away from any processed foods in the middle aisles, anything in a box or in a bag. (Except for my seaweed snacks, they're really good! They are packaged but organic, with only two ingredients.) My tips for freezer staples include keeping a supply of organic wild range chicken (all cuts), organic grass-fed beef, and a bag of wild caught salmon fillets in there at all times. You can thaw a tenderloin filet or salmon in a bowl of cold water for twenty minutes. A salmon dinner can be cooked in ten to twelve minutes, and that tenderloin filet can be seasoned and grilled in eight minutes flat using only a cast iron skillet. Whatever you do, don't shop hungry; it costs more, and you end up with stuff in your cart that you swear gremlins threw in when your head was turned.

Some tips for cooking from my kitchen to yours? Keeping it simple in my mind is the most important point. Too many widows and widowers say, "It's just me, I won't cook, maybe cheese and crackers or popcorn for dinner tonight." I was in the same boat, even though I cooked every night with Dave, and it was tough to get started in the beginning to know it was just for me. Every time I cooked after he was gone became a reminder he wasn't there watching me enjoy cooking. Even sitting and eating dinner alone was a challenge. A couple of times I sat at the table, thinking I was ready to eat, and just started sobbing, losing my desire to enjoy the meal I just cooked. It was okay though; it made great leftovers for the next day.

Pretty soon I realized if you don't eat well, you won't feel well, and you'll stay stuck not embracing life again. I created many new routines about cooking, from pre-prepping food for salads and meals, stocking things to always have on hand that can be thawed in twenty minutes to be cooked in a snap, and mentally getting over cooking for one. Getting used to life on my own was not easy, getting used to cooking for myself wasn't easy, but I knew if I went back to my old habits, I'd be right back up to an unhealthy weight. That alone was a good motivation for me to keep plugging forward.

I believe the change in what I was eating led to the elimination of many medications I was taking. I was on phentermine to lose weight, losartan for high blood pressure, metformin for pre-diabetes, lipitor for cholesterol, estradiol for hormone therapy, diazepan and sertraline for depression—they have all been eliminated from my life. Today I take only a few natural supplements, like fish oil, COQ10, and vitamins C and D. For natural pain relief I use arnica, turmeric, and some natural detox teas, like dandelion and licorice.

I open my kitchen cabinet and I still get a jolt to see nothing with a prescription label on it. In fact, the first thing I did the day after Dave died was to get a big garbage pail and toss every single one of his medications, all the cancer meds and everything else. This is a common occurrence I found out; a few of my widowed friends did the exact same thing.

I was married to a firefighter, who had probably ten cups of coffee a day for his entire life. Dave could have a cup of coffee after dinner, and it would put him to sleep immediately. I only had two cups in the morning back then, then I'd switch to organic herbal teas and a lot of water. I gave up my Keurig coffee maker after reading about moldy coffee, and also because of the food plan I was following religiously. Giving up coffee wasn't as bad as I thought it would be. A new habit has been my discovery of Organo King Coffee and drinking my one cup in the morning which doesn't give me the jitters like regular coffee does and is actually good for you. It's made with ganoderma mushrooms, one of the oldest used in Chinese herbalism. Some studies show ganoderma can boost immunity, fight fatigue, relieve stress and my favorite—help the aging process.

My energy levels are through the roof with these easy lifestyle changes; just ask my classmates at the Functional Medicine Coaching Academy and my friends!

Step 2: Incorporate Movement Into Every Day

Have you heard? Sitting is the new smoking.

Most people think they must spend hours and hours working out in a gym. I'm here to tell you that's not true. Movement can be just about anything—except sitting! Actually, you can sit, but maybe use that time to do chair yoga, chair dancing, or just stretch your arms to the ceiling.

Movement is so key to living longer, looking better, and feeling better. I can also tell you from experience it helps with brain fog, also known as "widow fog." Widow fog is very, very real. Trust me on this one, I looked it up.

There are so many ways to move. One idea is to join an exercise class, not only for the movement, but also to meet new like-minded people in a safe environment. I worked out with a trainer at my local gym for many years, the YMCA, and it has helped me get away from the all-consuming grief, especially in the first year. I never missed a date in all those years, and it was my motivation to get my butt to the gym. My trainer was my accountability coach, and remains so even after the pandemic when we went virtual.

Gardening counts as movement too and can be therapeutic nurturing a garden to life. Another good thing is feeling the stretch the next morning after using muscles that are quite different than the usual ones used. Cleaning the house is another good use of energy, from dusting to vacuuming to washing floors—all good for the mind and body. I actually work up a sweat when I vacuum!

Start slow, crawl, walk, run if you want! Just start moving, it's so important to help you feel better. Just walk, for example—it's free. Park at the furthest spot in the parking lot, take the stairs, pace around your house, just get moving.

There are a number of smartphone apps which can help you monitor, track, and get motivated with a gentle nudge (or kick in the arse) to get moving. One of my favorite tools is my Oura Ring. It tracks everything from sleep, to temperature, to activity, to my body's recovery to face the next day. Seeing the results of my efforts on the Oura Ring tracker gave me confidence to continue my health and fitness journey. To this day, it's the first thing I check every single morning.

There are a number of free exercise apps out there too, from grief yoga, Gaiam Yoga, to "7 minute workouts" to "Map My Run" which I use all the time for my walks, even beach strolls. Exercise to a schedule, make a date with yourself, put it on your calendar to get up and get out. Anything that can be measured can be improved, as Dr. Habib told me. Exercise has helped to soften the grief, plus it helped me to feel better physically. It was nice to wake up and see my life and attitude improving most days.

One Sunday, my local YMCA even had a jiu jitsu class for women in self-defense. It was the first time in my life I threw a man to the ground over my shoulder—what a thrill! At the gym I took yoga classes, strength classes, stretching, and even high intensity workouts. It was a great way to meet new people in a safe place. There are many free online courses, especially lots for yoga, mostly all for free on YouTube. Yoga is a favorite of mine, not only for the flexibility benefits but the breathing benefits as well.

After Dave died, I heard about massage being good grief therapy. I couldn't deal with a new man in my life, but I definitely could deal with a regular masseuse! The first time I had a Thai Massage it was incredible. I remember saying to my masseuse, "That was the most incredible yoga session ever, and you did all the work!" He said, "That's why they call it Lazy Man's yoga." I like deep tissue massages also.. Massage is a great help for grief; you can even find "gentle touch" massage specifically for grief support. I try to schedule a massage and alternate it with a Thai Massage as often as I can, wherever I am. It's funny, because when I was married, I rarely had a massage, mostly only if we were on a cruise ship that had a spa.

There are so many ways to move but one of my most favorite is a beach walk. The beach is great for grounding and healing. Dr. Jimerson told me the magnesium in the ocean water helps to heal. What better reason to spend time on the beach with your toes in the sand and wading in the water? A sedentary lifestyle leads to obesity, plus couch potatoes are not that attractive.

When should you move? For me, mornings are best. I like starting the day with a walk with friends especially, a yoga session, or the gym. I love this saying: "Win the morning, win the day." Move five minutes every hour, set a schedule, make a date. Just do it!

It was also good to have a reason to get out of bed in the morning. In the beginning, when my eyes opened up and I realized I was alone, it hit me hard. Our mornings together were the best part of the day with Dave.

Step 3: Improve Sleep

When Queen Elizabeth lost her beloved Prince Philip, much was written about widows and sleep disruption. The world was genuinely worried about her health as well. Studies have shown the surviving spouse can suffer from sleep challenges which then leads down a slippery slope of depression, anxiety, impaired immune system, and overall poorer physical health. I know my sleep suffered a LOT. I'd wake up often in the middle of the night, and just lie there for hours, thinking about how sad life was, how sad I was, and how alone I felt.

Sleep is so important! We spend almost a third of our life sleeping. Unfortunately, one of the first things they prescribe to widows and widowers are sleeping pills; the second thing they often prescribe is antidepressants. Resist! They are only masking the problem; sedation does not equal good sleep (and the next day may cause fogginess, which we certainly don't need more of). It's not the restorative, healing kind of sleep you need. Melatonin supplements may help on a temporary basis, for example if you're just returning from a long trip and may have jet lag. Otherwise, no aids should be needed.

Sleep is a great grief buster too. The three Rs of sleep are recovery, rejuvenation, and reduction—of anxiety, stress, and grief. If you're well-rested, you can deal with stress and anxiety better and it helps you have more strength to get through the days alone. An added bonus of good sleep: weight management. Studies show that overweight people generally are not getting enough good sleep. People who are well-rested also tend to be seen as more attractive, as other studies have shown.

Good sleep is the key to longevity by restoring the immune system, helping you recover from daily exercise, and even weight regulation. If you want to live to be older than one hundred, like I do, then good sleep is a MUST. Good sleep helps with healing, wellness, longevity, and even learning. Poor sleep can lead to many disorders, like high blood pressure, depression, and even obesity. Not to mention the bags under the eyes.

The trinity of survival is drinking, eating, and sleeping. We live in a culture that doesn't understand the importance of sleep and its impact on your health and wellbeing. If you don't drink, you will die. If you don't eat, you will die. If you don't sleep, you will die. Proper sleep is absolutely critical when caring for yourself.

Here are some of my tips for getting that good night's sleep:

- Sleeping in a dark cold room. My thermostat is set to sixty-seven degrees, following recommendations for temperatures between sixty-five and sixty-eight. You can actually see your breath in my bedroom!
- Dark and cold improve the two S's – Sleep and Sex only.
- No TV or email or phone at least an hour before bed— preferably two hours. This could be causing your middle of the night wake-up. (Mine used to be between two and four in the morning.)

- Stop food and alcohol two hours before sleep time.
- Try to go to bed at the same time every night. I shoot for 10:00 p.m. and strive for seven to eight hours.
- Watch your caffeine intake. I found that if I have anything after 12:00 noon, I'll be up in the middle of the night for hours. I go to sleep within minutes just fine, but I don't stay asleep. I learned why; it's about the half-life of caffeine which is five hours to get half of the caffeine out of your system. This means if you have your last cup at noon, at 5:00 p.m. it will be half gone, and then at 10:00 p.m. it will be all out of your system until the next day.
- Try a cup of calming Chamomile tea an hour before bedtime—they call it Sleepy Time tea for a reason.
- Turn off all your electronic devices two to three hours before bed. There are glasses you can buy to block blue light as well, the light that keeps you up at night.

Part of the aftermath of deep grief is sleeplessness. As my health improved, so did my sleep. Now, if I am restless during the night, sometimes I'll listen to a sleep story through my Calm app, or practice a guided Yoga Nidra meditation with my airpods on. Keith Urban, one of my favorite artists, actually wrote a sleep song which is on the Calm app.

One of my favorite breathing exercises to fall asleep is called four-seven-eight, also known as Relaxing Breath, according to Dr. Weil. It's a natural depressant for your nervous system, slows down your heart, and helps you fall asleep in seconds. It quiets the part of the brain where stress hangs out. Here's how you do it: Breathe in for a count of four, hold your breath for a count of seven, and exhale for a count of eight. Two or three times doing this, and it puts me right to sleep! If I happen to wake up in the middle of the night boiling over from a hot flash (do they EVER go away?), this is also what I do then.

Sunshine is another key factor to sleeping well. Sachin Patel (Living

Proof Institute) was a proponent of being out in the sun for ten minutes in the morning, at sunset, and at noon, preferably naked. Seriously. I had to chuckle at this suggestion because I used to live on a golf course right next to the cart path on the fourth hole. I imagined the Wednesday Men's League driving by in their golf carts and yelling, "Put it back on!" Not to mention it's probably illegal in most states.

Sunlight in your eyes in the morning sets your biological clock to say, "Hey World, I'm awake and it's morning." Noon sunlight is when you get the best levels of vitamin D—the sun vitamin—which helps with your immune system and your overall health. Watching the sunset is great for relaxation and calming and getting your body and mind ready to call it a day.

Step 4: Meditate to Reduce Stress

Meditation? Not my cup of tea, or so I thought. I had a hard time becoming a believer (like many people I've talked to). I tried! Could not quiet the constant chattering of the monkey brain and didn't quite know how to breathe—not to mention I didn't even know about the tremendous benefits of breathwork and meditation. Speaking of breathwork, did you know your body could kill you in four short minutes by just not breathing? When I was diagnosed with chronic stress, my research kept pointing back to one thing: you must meditate to reduce that stress, the biggest and most dangerous issue Dr. Habib uncovered.

Meditation has now become an amazing and much needed addition to my life after Dave died. As my body healed, it was time to work on the spirit. There's one guideline that says it takes doing something for thirty days in a row to make it a permanent habit, and I will tell you it is so true, especially for me. I dabbled with the Calm app years ago, but never really made it a habit. Next, I discovered Deepak Chopra and Oprah's 21-day meditation series, and that was just okay but didn't stick with me. YouTube was next, and that's how

I discovered Wayne Dyer and his "I am Enough" meditations.

I have learned so much about breathwork since that one day in Dr. Jimerson's office when he taught me how to belly breathe. Here's what he had me do: put one hand on your chest, and one hand on your stomach while focusing on breathing deeply through your belly. Many people don't realize how much of a shallow breather they might be until you learn how to deep breathe through your belly. Meditation classes also taught me different types of breathing as well, helping during anxiety attacks and even temper tantrums. Here's another easy example: inhale for a count of four, exhale for a count of eight, it's called "double time breathing." This was a major step in learning to deal with anxiety and grief without medication, just deep breathing.

Emily Fletcher and her book *Stress Less, Accomplish More* and her online ZIVA course was the turning point into helping forge this into a habit that is now automatic every morning. I finally got over the feeling that maybe meditation was just not for me! I learned that so many people feel the same way.

Did you know that a brief meditation can offer rest that's five times deeper than sleep? Plus, it's an antidote to stress and anxiety. Stress is classified as being a reaction to something happening right now, while anxiety is classed as a reaction to something that may happen in the future. Stress can cause anxiety, anxiety can cause stress, and both get in the way of overcoming grief and embracing life again. The first couple of times I meditated, it was very emotional. Things would come up by surprise, and I didn't know from where, but all of a sudden I'd be crying. The combination of meditation and learning how to breathe was essential in helping me work through my feelings of grief and taking the time to honor my loss and gain clarity about how I needed to move forward. Plus, it helped me visualize and manifest what I really wanted in order to be happy again.

I mix up my daily meditations with Vishen Lakiani's six phase meditation which focuses on compassion, gratitude, forgiveness, future vision, the perfect day, and ending with a blessing. Wayne Dyer is pretty amazing as well, and YouTube has many of his guided meditations to follow. Dr. Joe Dispenza has been another influence on my meditation practice especially after reading his book "Becoming Supernatural."

Give meditation a try, the ability to reduce stress, anxiety, and calm the grief down is well studied and it really works. Start small, start breathing, and just sit quietly with yourself. It helped me find calmness and reduce the stress and anxiety I was feeling. Meditation is the art of being present, and when I mastered being present in the moment, this helped me heal. But I say give it a try for only thirty days. It can be as little as three minutes a day. It can be guided or unguided. Sit with your breathing to music, or simply gaze into outer space with your eyes closed.

I can just imagine the look of disbelief and then the smile on Dave's face if he saw me meditating to the sounds of the universe and losing track of time and space!

Step 5: Increase Laughter!

Smiling and laughing has a positive effect on your wellbeing, not to mention makes you more approachable and more attractive— ten times better than a sad face. Did you know a smile is our first facial expression after birth? So what if it's usually caused by gas in a baby—it's still contagious! I remember asking a fellow widow how she got through the days of her grief. She told me she tried to find something to smile about every single day. It really does work. I was feeling guilty at first for smiling, but then I realized it felt good to embrace humor again, and it was okay to laugh again even though it took me at least six months.

The first time I laughed out loud, it startled me. The sound was so strange I had to do a double take wondering what that noise was. It was me! From a physical perspective, laughing releases the feel-good chemical endorphins, and decreases the stress hormone, cortisol. It's a great boost to your immune system too.

Therapy helped me in many ways, including getting over this newfound guilt I had of being happy. When I finally felt ready to find a good grief therapist, it was about six months later, and it was so worth it. Your typical grief counseling group wasn't what I thought I needed or wanted. Hospice had a number of suggestions for me, but none resonated. When I found my therapist, we immediately connected on a personal level, and I felt I could really open up to her. She helped me realize laughter was not about running away from grief, but actually about overcoming the guilt of laughing. It's about knowing your loved one is gone and not able to laugh with you, but wanting you to keep going on living.

My therapist cried with me as we both talked through the stories about Dave, making me miss him terribly as we talked through my grieving process. She tracked where I was at and how I was feeling during each meeting. Do you know what the most powerful question was that she asked me? "Do you hold any regrets?" It stopped me in my tracks for a second, just a second, and the answer was a resounding *no*—there wasn't anything left unsaid between Dave and me.

After Dave died, I started writing about stories and memories that came pouring out. In fact, this book began as a journal! I kept all the napkins from plane trips and restaurants, the Post-it Notes, the handwritten notes on any available scrap, and even the original journal book. Writing down these memories was an incredible way to process and deal with my grief.

Journaling is a great way to reconnect with memories, and another good way to make you smile and laugh. Dave and I had tons of funny stories from our travels, his life in the fire department, and from my career. I also have a gratitude journal which I write in every morning and evening.

One of the things I wanted to do was share and write about experiences in my journal that I thought Dave would love, even if he couldn't be there. I held two golf memorials in his honor, with benefits going to the Youth Hockey Scholarship Fund (one of our loves was hockey). We became the biggest sponsor to the scholarship fund—what an honor that is and Dave would have been so happy at this knowledge. I wrote about this event the first year and the second year in my journal. Many of his friends could sense his presence on the golf course, especially when we had a "Hit the Ball into the Water for Dave" contest!

Dave was honored at three walls as a Line of Duty Death, and I have volunteered at these memorials to help others get through the most difficult times. If I can make them smile for a brief moment, putting their sadness aside, then it makes my heart full.

Through the navigation of my grief process, I tried to find other things that would make me smile and laugh. I watched *Major League* the other night for the tenth time at least, and just smiled and chuckled all the way through. I am probably one of the last people who still like to read a newspaper the old fashioned way, in my hands at the kitchen table. I have an affliction; I cannot buy a newspaper and not read it from front to back. The best reason for me is to get to the funnies, my reward for finishing.

The latest way to connect with friends and family is for Zoom happy hours. Even after the pandemic ends, I think this trend will continue. My friend got me on Facetime for the first time in my life, and I got him on Zoom. What a wonderful way to be with old friends and family from around the world.

There's an app for that! There really are a lot for making you smile. Check out "Laugh your App Off" for a joke a day. Another great idea is to find funny friends. You know that friend you have that makes you laugh at the silliest things? They are worth their weight in gold. I have a few friends like that, especially my friend Anne. We can get together once a year (we are very far apart and in different countries) and it doesn't matter how long it's been, we're smiling and laughing within minutes. If you don't have any funny friends in your life, hang around children; nothing is more infectious than a child laughing. Dave and

I loved our roles as Aunt and Uncle to the many children in our lives.

Mark Twain has a great quote, "Against the assault of laughter, nothing can stand."

Step 6: Develop Healthy Relationships

My twelve fellow classmates from the Coaching Academy always liked my motto of "militant positivity." Thinking right and positive was so important for me to overcome my tremendous grief. Talk right to yourself at all times and be kind to yourself. Your words matter. How you talk to yourself is the most important conversation you will have every single day.

Other ideas and practices I embraced included my gratitude journal. I write in it almost every day and every night. It only takes minutes. First thing in the morning, I set an intention and affirmations for the day. At night, thinking back on my day helps me remember the things for which I am grateful. Some days it was as simple as a fine meal cooked for only myself, with the table set and the candles lit. Even then, sitting alone at dinner wasn't always positive, many times I'd dissolve into a puddle of tears after one bite. Gratitude can help to decrease depression. One day I received a letter of gratitude totally out of the blue from an old neighbor. It simply said, "I'm grateful to have known you." Very powerful stuff.

Unsubscribe to negative people in your life. This goes for friends AND family! Friends who criticize you or are envious of you are not good for your mental state. You'll have enough challenges without the negativity. The first thing I did was to "unsubscribe" to the negative people around me. It was liberating to say the least. Negative people will discourage you and they will try to drag you down with them to the dark side. As Robert Tew once said, "Don't let negative and toxic people rent space in your head. Raise the rent and kick them out."

The top three traits I look for in the people who I want to spend time with are:

1. First, give me the freedom to grieve. You never know when it's going to pop up.
2. Second, trust in a friend to be kind and show empathy.
3. Third, have respect for muddled brains and have my back as my life evolves and morphs into Life Part 2.

My girlfriends around me in the neighborhood were priceless to have by my side. We were really close, and they were always on hand at a moment's notice to cry with me on the front porch, grill with me on the back deck, or sit in the kitchen over a glass of wine (or two). I have to say, they were instrumental in my picking these important top three traits for anyone close to me, especially empathy.

Jim Rohn says in his book *Art of Exceptional Living*, "You are the average of the five people you spend the most time with." So choose wisely who you spend time with.

When I moved to Sarasota, I was all by myself, no friends or family. Do you know what's scarier than skydiving when you're afraid of heights? Trying to find new friends in a new city and starting a new life as a solo adventurer. It's hard to be part of a couple for so many years with mostly couple friends. We lived in a community of families and couples and not many singles at all. This is the primary reason for me picking up, moving, and starting over. There was nothing really for a single female to do in our lovely golf community. Plus, it was time for me to find not only a new house but a new "home."

Widowhood Sucks, especially after 50! That's the name of my "Meetup" group which has been an adventure. Meetup is a way for anyone to start a group for people of like interests, get together at varied events, and make new friends. I started it to meet new people and get out into the social scene again. It's up to over one hundred members, and my first kiss came from someone in that group!

There are many different Facebook groups to join, all geared toward widowhood. Simply search "widowhood" and you'll find them. Many of them will ask a question about your partner's date of death, so they make sure there are no "lurkers" in the group, and to keep the group safe and secure.

Maybe try to find a common local group. Perhaps it's a bereavement support group. There's a wonderful book I read, *The Turquoise Table*, which described another way to meet people. Simply put a table out in your front yard, have a cup of coffee, and you'd be amazed at who might just join you for coffee.

Dating, on the other hand, is kind of weird. I couldn't even say the word DATING with a straight face, let alone think about sex! I discovered men and women process things differently. Men who I've talked to tend to get over things more quickly. From a couple of widowers I talked to, it was a mere six months. For me, it didn't even cross my mind until a year and a half went by, and I was kissed so unexpectedly and passionately that my shoes melted right off my feet. From then on, it crossed my mind a lot!

According to statistics, in 2018, about 11.69 million widows were living in the United States, whereas the number of widowers was at about 3.4 million. In Canada there's about 1.9 million, with 75% of them widows. It's funny, but men usually start looking for another woman between six and nine months after being widowed, get married, and then they're not in that widowed status anymore. I met a twice widowed gentleman in Florida, and he waited a short three months before he was dating again. Women I've talked to normally don't even think about dating for one to two years and sometimes never. Maybe it's because women feel stuck or frozen, like they're wearing concrete boots. I've been told other comments, like, "He was the best, don't need the rest!" For me I was ready after about a year and a half, still feeling like I had a lot of love to give, and still wanting to "do life" with a fun partner again.

10 Tips for Dating a Widow is an article sent to me by my friend. It is well written and very true. You can also find *10 Tips for Dating a Widower* online. There are so many great resources online, and the content is amazing.

Going through class with the coaching academy exposed me to a whole new community. A new tribe of friends, acquaintances, and mentors all focused on the same thing—wellness. Within this new group, we became accountability partners to each other. It helped me tremendously as I neared the end of going through the firsts and lasts without Dave. They also helped to overcome the *overwhelm* of so many things on my plate and focus on doing just one thing at a time, like finish the book!

It's a great idea to take a course, and it's great to meet new people this way. Other ideas might be to take a cooking course, a language course, or even a basket weaving course! Someone asked me how they could travel more, and my response was—just buy a ticket. Go ahead and create new memories. Your partner would want you to live life, thrive, and not give up. I know that this is what Dave wanted very much for me.

Step 7: Discover New Purpose

After I healed myself physically, it was now time to expand my horizons and discover how I could find new purpose in what I affectionately call "Life Part 2." It started with an email from Sachin Patel (Living Proof Institute) about becoming a Functional Medicine Certified Health Coach. When I read that email, I got goosebumps. Going back to school for another year reminded me so much of Dave. He was with me through all my courses that I took over the years, even going back to finish my bachelor's degree at age fifty. He was my biggest backer and supporter following me and my love of education. He preserved in me my love of learning. When I enrolled in the Coaching Academy, it put a new bounce in my step. I was going to learn something completely new and different, perhaps giving me a reason to jump out of bed every morning, and you're never too old to become a learner.

When the student is ready, the teacher will appear, and sure enough, Mahnaz appeared. Mahnaz Malik was our "course facilitator" at the coaching academy, but she will forever be "teacher" in my mind. I cannot stress enough what a tremendous influence Mahnaz has had on my life-changing transformation through the Coaching Academy, and also helping me to get over the grief of losing Dave. The twelve classmates we spent a year with became our "Tribe of Coaches," and each of us has a vision to help the world get well. This tribe is a support network, accountability partners to each other, and a really great group of people, all thrown together, by chance, with Mahnaz as the leader.

My purpose came to me after graduating as a wellness coach. At the same time, I realized the journal I started was actually coming to life as a book. The twelve chapters and titles came to me, and even though it has changed drastically (for the better) from the first edition, all chapters remained. Friends and family read the opening chapters, and they encouraged me to carry on! Everyone I told my story to was inspired, both with the stories about my health transformation and then my life transformation.

Give yourself permission to live again; you deserve it. Dave was more worried about me than he was about his impending death. It was hard, but being ready to embrace life again gave me the strength to find my new life's purpose.

There are many national widows' groups like Soaring Spirits and the Modern Widows Club, lots on Facebook, Grief Yoga on the web, and many more resources when you're ready to start something new. I have an idea for holding widow retreats, talking about nutrition, cooking, yoga, long walks on the beach, and resources for widows and widowers. There's a lot out there to discover.

Paul Denniston, founder of "Grief Yoga," explores moving into purpose in his classes. It's good to find new purpose to get you out of bed in the morning, instead of just waiting for your time on earth to run out. Besides, it can be fun! It's nice to laugh and smile again, and believe me, the memories never go away of the time spent together with Dave, but it's cool for me to know I'll honor our past life with the making of new memories and having new adventures.

*"Grief is not a disorder, a disease, or a sign of weakness.
It is an emotional, physical, and spiritual necessity, the price you
pay for love. The only cure for grief is to grieve."*

—Rabbi Earl Grollman

CHAPTER 8

Manifesting with Velocity

*O*nce I healed my body from the inside physically, I started wondering, *what's next?* It's important to know, and this was always in the back of my mind, that Dave gave me permission to embrace life and wanted me to be happy again if and when I was ready. We talked about it during his last six months of life. By the way—it was exactly six months from diagnosis to prognosis—how do they know? Good data and statistics, I learned.

My classmates at the Coaching Academy (especially Derek) told me I was the epitome of "Manifesting with Velocity," and it was really true! During my meditations I would think about my dreams and desires for the next year, and one after another, they came to reality.

I felt like the rest of my life was starting over and ahead of me. I was ready to embrace life again. About a year and a half after Dave died, the first and biggest change I made was to relocate. As scary as it was, it was time to move on and leave South Carolina. The community where Dave and I spent twenty years was full of couples and families. Not really a good place for social activities as a single. I went from being part of a couple which was very safe, to being a solo female which was awkward as hell. After a year and a half alone in our old neighborhood, I felt like the proverbial third wheel. "Let's make sure we ask Marie, the widow, to join us for dinner, or a play, or some other event." They were all sincere requests, so well meaning, and I did love it at first. After a while it didn't feel right anymore. I wanted to start to find my own way through the next chapter of my life, and I was ready.

Every move and every decision is hard. It's scary to do, but I put on my big girl pants and did it anyway. I never looked back or regretted any decision I made all by myself, without my partner Dave by my side to lend an ear.

The "7 Steps to Healing After Loss" helped me to regain confidence in myself and rediscover my loves as both an adventurer and as a learner. Florida had beckoned me since I was a teenager when I went to Fort Lauderdale with friends over spring break. Over the years, Dave and I had looked at property there for a second home, mostly on the Atlantic Ocean side. After discovering Sarasota and the Gulf Coast side of Florida the year before, it became my desire to learn more. An Airbnb condo came available on the white crystal sand beach at Siesta Key where I spent a glorious month. So I packed up my car, locked up the house, and headed south. I wasn't really sure yet what my plans were, but I was ready for the adventure with an open mind, healed body, and calm spirit.

Siesta Key is a beautiful beach and in 2020 was ranked the #1 Beach in the US by TripAdvisor. White, quartz-crystal sand beckoned me every morning. I'd go for a walk every day, about three to four miles, then sit on the sand and write. This condo was pretty special. Because of the time of year and the location of the unit at the end of the building, I saw the sun rise and the sun set each and every day! There was only one other place I experienced this, and it was on the beach at a place called the Atlantic resort where Dave and I stayed a few times on Daytona Beach.

As much as I loved being by the ocean every day and night on Siesta Key, I found myself spending most nights in the city of Sarasota, about a twenty-minute ride away. There were so many restaurants to try, and live bands playing at a lot of different venues. The city beckoned me every night.

It wasn't as bad as I thought it was going to be, in a strange new place, not knowing anyone, but I was ready. I was also happy with my decision to leave my house (and my comfort zone) in South Carolina. Dave and I had spent a lot of good years in that neighborhood, making many friends, both golfers and non-golfers. We loved it there.

I started to meet new people right away through my girlfriends' groups on Meetup which felt really good. I was letting friends back in my life, new and old. Christmas and New Years were spent with the girls, many of them widows, at wonderful restaurants having wonderful holiday dinners. Feeling good about myself helped me smile again and made me grateful for the strength and will to embrace life again.

One day after about a month on Siesta Key, with a lot of reflection during my solo beach walks, through meditation and self-discovery, I said to myself, "What are you waiting for?" Just do it! Pack up, sell the house, and move. I won't lie and tell you it was easy—it wasn't. Lots of times I questioned my motives and self-doubt crept in, especially since I would be leaving behind so many close girlfriends. It was hard not having a partner to talk things through with. Dave and I always discussed everything at length, including any purchase over $500!

I was truly thinking I'd just go to Florida for just a couple of months, especially to get away from the Christmas holidays and not have to deal with another year of memories alone. Going through those firsts and lasts in year one was really draining. You didn't know how you were going to react, what emotions would bubble up to the surface, and whether you'd be alone or in public when they did strike.

A glorious and rare unfurnished three-bedroom condo became available for rent near downtown Sarasota. It was important to me to find an unfurnished condo because I wanted my own kitchen stuff and cookware with me. I wanted to work on this first book and my budding thoughts of a cookbook. Most condos in Florida are furnished because it's such a rental and Airbnb destination. That same day, I rented the condo, overlooking Sarasota Bay, signing a one-year lease. I hadn't sold my house yet, but that was okay, as I knew it would go quickly. I only signed a one-year lease, because I had no idea where life was going to take me in a year. I also felt that after all I went through in making repairs to the house and finding someone to do the work (especially as a single female), there was really no need for me to own property again.

I made a phone call to someone I knew was interested in buying my house, and we had a deal within a week. The phone call with the decision to buy came as I was shopping for groceries, and the holler I let out made a few heads turn! The timing was perfect, as the new owners were headed south to Florida to see friends. We made the deal official and signed the papers at lunch in a restaurant off the highway. Let my new life begin.

I graduated as a Functional Medicine Certified Health Coach after passing the final live coaching oral exam while in the middle of the move to Florida. Dave would have been proud; after all, he was with me for all my educational endeavors and successes before. This was a great moment for me, and I wished he was with me to help celebrate.

During that time, I was so fortunate to have my dear friend Brooke help me pack up the house and supervise the movers, and she sold a ton of excess stuff for me. She also came down to Florida to help set up the condo and move me in.

The day I left the house in South Carolina was sad—mixed emotions flooded through me. Thinking about the timeline in that house, Dave and I had really only enjoyed this place for three short months before he fell ill and faced the end of his life, changing mine forever at the same time.

I had one last flashback before leaving the house of Dave being wheeled out of the bedroom on a gurney the Sunday morning he died, headed to the funeral home. We tucked a golf ball in his pocket, I took a lock of his hair for a keepsake, and we lowered the Canadian flag to half-staff in front of the house. The funeral home left behind a single red rose on his pillow after they took Dave away. When I opened the closed bedroom door and saw that single red rose, I broke down and sobbed and sobbed. A beautiful single red rose which held the power to make me collapse on the bedroom floor.

Continuing with the major life changes, a month after I moved into the condo, I decided to retire from my thirty-year career in technology. It wasn't a snap decision; Dave and I prepared and worked toward this for a couple of years before he died. Actually picking the date and going through with it was quite a huge decision and another scary one. It was tough to make this decision without talking it through with my life coach, Dave, since the planning for this retirement day had started with him. But I did it and never looked back (even as the global pandemic you might have heard about crept closer and closer over the next two months).

I laugh nowadays and joke that I don't know how I ever had time to work.

Friends, new and old, supported me and had my back as I rediscovered my purpose of how I wanted to live the rest of my life. As the book emerged, I began sharing my thoughts and new dreams with my smart friends Linda and Cyndy. They all loved the first version of the book, and supported my decision to move to Sarasota in the first place. I got out of my comfort zone and made the dreams bigger than my fears.

Someone once said, "Your comfort zone is where dreams go to die."

My sense of adventure and willingness to try new things and see new places was reborn. I had no desire to just survive—I wanted to THRIVE—especially with longevity running in my family. I was willing to take a risk. I started by trying small ones, like going out to dinner by myself. You'll never know who you might meet. My "attitude of gratitude" helped me get through each new day, by being thankful for all that was happening around me.

After retiring, I no longer had excuses to not finish this book.

The first draft finally got finished a month later, and I remember flinging open the balcony doors and screaming at the top of my lungs over Sarasota Bay:

"Dave, we did it! We wrote a book!"

PART 3

The Beginning

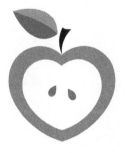

CHAPTER 9

The Ashes are Scattered, Now What?

One morning, the doors flew open on Dave's armoire in our old house in South Carolina. This is where I kept the scattering tube with his ashes. I remember yelling, "I know, I know, I'll get right on the scattering!" I couldn't help but think this was a sign for me to march on and get going on "Life Part 2." It's what he wanted, and I was ready.

We celebrated Dave with a golf memorial at the course where we lived. I wanted it to be special, and it was. It was a perfect day, family and friends came in from all over the US and Canada, had a fun eighteen holes of golf, and grilled ribeye's—Dave's favorite steak. We even had a few fun contests, such as hitting it into the water on one of his nemesis holes; he hit a lot of balls into that hazard on the 12th hole over the twenty years of golf at our course.

The ashes were scattered on one of the ponds at our golf course during his golf memorial. Dave wanted to be with all his lost balls in the water. Seriously. He said this to everyone for years before he died.

My love of learning has been with me my whole life. I went to college after graduating high school, working full time and attending classes in the evenings. My Associates Degree was in Human Resource Management. At age fifty, I declared one day to Dave that it was time to finish my bachelor's degree, so off I went to night school.

Now, I was ready to learn something new about myself, my grief, and how I could start healing and figure out Life Part Two.

I went back to school through the Functional Medicine Coaching Academy (FMCA) for a program to become a Functional Medicine Certified Health Coach. One of the first assignments was to take a free survey online. It's called the VIA survey, and I think everyone should take this test! (https://www.viacharacter.org/).

Lo and behold my top five strengths are:

1. Humor (didn't know this when I came up with the title of this book!)
2. Kindness
3. Gratitude
4. Appreciation of Beauty and Excellence
5. Creativity

This is what my strengths mean to me: Humor gets me through life one day at a time and makes me smile. Kindness to friends, family, and strangers makes me smile. Kindness helps me to focus on others and not so much on my pain and loss. Gratitude is an amazing strength and helps me get through each and every day by keeping a gratitude journal. Gratitude helps me find something to smile about every day by focusing on what I have today and what Dave helped build for us. Appreciation of Beauty and Excellence in my environment, travels, and this world makes me smile. Creativity is helping me write this book which makes me smile! Now if I can only get my lesser strength "Perseverance" to rise up to the challenge, I'll get more of my creative endeavors finished.

The FMCA year-long course focused on five specific pillars of "Wellness." Wellness is the following five foundational pillars of the Functional Medicine Matrix that we learned about.

1. Sleep and Relaxation
2. Exercise and Movement
3. Nutrition
4. Stress
5. Relationships

During the year-long program of coaching and being coached on these Wellness pillars, a lifelong bond was created with my fellow classmates. It's a global group from Berlin to Australia, US, Saudi Arabia, India, and Canada. We call ourselves "A Tribe of Coaches." Our leader, the Magnificent Mahnaz Malik, is responsible for helping each one of us connect to our purpose and help to transform our lives and others with our coaching passions. Each week we coached and were coached on the pillars of wellness using our own personal experiences and feelings, along with case study examples. The course was very well done, and so enlightening.

I was overwhelmed at the time with everything on my plate, still working and still suffering from lingering "widow brain fog." When I got that way, nothing got done, and I end up pacing in circles. It was an ongoing theme for me during my coaching sessions. At one of my office hour visits with Mahnaz, we got to talking about everything going on. She said to me—or should I say she pulled it out of me— *finish the book*. It had to be the number one priority, because it was the catalyst to everything else.

Talk about boiling the ocean down to one single statement.

Our tribe of coaches are all chasing our dreams and new purposes in life together, and without this tribe, this book would not have gotten off the ground in the first place. We've held each other accountable for reaching our goals and keeping our dreams in focus. The Coaching Academy helped me find my new purpose in life, helped deal with the grief of losing Dave, and taught me how to help others by coaching. Classes have helped me reflect, learn more about my mind, body, spirit, and move forward from the tremendous grief of losing Dave. It has been truly life-changing.

I want to spread the word about Functional Medicine far and wide. Sachin Patel (Founder of LPI) who suggested I join the FMCA program in the first place, says, "The Doctor of the Future is the Patient," and I truly believe that wise saying. I was realizing more and more every day that I was the captain of my own ship. It was up to me to make the right choices, choose the right path, and get on with the business of living life.

One thing I wonder about all the time is if I could have done better to help Dave with his cancer, especially cooking for Dave if I knew then what I know now about diet, nutrition, cancer, and functional medicine. Dr. Jimerson did give me some advice to try—like CBD cream, oil, juices—and it did help Dave a little bit. During our last cruise, I had him try a green juice (kale, celery, parsley, cilantro), because he wasn't eating much by then. He said, "Yuck, this tastes like grass!" So much for that experiment!

All of this has led me to my purpose for "Life Part 2" which is to help widows and widowers learn to live well, laugh more, and love again. This was a new beginning for my life, a life where Dave now lived in my heart instead of by my side in the kitchen.

The ashes are scattered. Now pass the asparagus.

CHAPTER 10

Cooking with a Side of Kleenex

*S*o there I was, cooking pasta for myself the first time, never feeling so alone. As the tears were flowing out of my eyes, I blew my nose and raised a glass of wine to the heavens and said, "Thank you, Dave, you let me cook and experiment on you for thirty years!"

The first shopping trip after Dave died brought me to tears. I was in the supermarket alone for the first time (Dave always did the shopping) buying ONE chicken breast, buying ONE filet, and ONE piece of salmon, and it made me realize I was in this alone and I better just suck it up, cook for myself, and get on with getting and staying healthy. I ran into one of my neighbors in the supermarket that day; she saw me in tears and joined me. There we were, standing in the meat section, bawling our eyes out.

Now, when I grill salmon or steak, if I'm alone, I'll eat half for dinner and the rest for lunch the next day. Freezing my favorite dishes like chicken champagne thighs or crispy chicken legs works too. It was a whole new cooking world opened up to me, and I was determined to make the best of it. After all, cooking is my passion. It makes me smile to get creative, and I love cooking for others.

Mom left this earth the same year as Dave, on December 7, 2018, to bake cookies for Dad and Dave in heaven. In her obituary, I wrote: *"Mom instilled in all of us a love of cooking, and for some of us a love of baking."* I was never a baker (and didn't want sweets in the house anyway because neither of us could resist). I said for years that I felt Mom was put on this earth to feed people. She cooked dinner for the family (and straggler friends and neighbors) every single night, and every Sunday was the famous sauce that cooked all day long. All of my sisters and brothers have different versions of Mom's "Sunday" sauce. Dinner time growing up was always together around the kitchen table, for ten people every single night. The family grew with girlfriends and boyfriends who became spouses and then they had children. Sunday dinner became a sit down pasta dinner (usually about two or three in the afternoon) for twenty to twenty-four people every single Sunday. All of this in a small 1,000 square foot house where everyone congregated around the kitchen and dining room.

Growing up, food fights were inevitable, especially when we were left alone. One of the funniest stories included green beans, tomatoes, and sausage all stewed in one big pot—usually one of our favorites. That evening Mom and Dad went out, unfortunately the beans were not cooked, and an all-out food fight ensued. Luckily, we were all very good at cleaning up and hiding the messes we made when left alone. Another funny story involved a BIG pot of mashed potatoes which none of us were particularly fond of. It was probably due to the monotonous grind of peeling ten pounds of potatoes, cutting them up, and cooking them until mush. When we cleaned up after dinner with mashed potatoes, our favorite part was scooping the rest of them out of the pot using our hands (the pot was huge) and throwing it into the garbage. This one time, in winter, my brother was inspired to take that handful of mashed potatoes and throw them at the detached garage out back! My dad was curious for months why this one snowball wasn't melting when spring came. Little did he realize it was a "forever snowball" made out of mashed potatoes which turned hard as cement.

Mom was 100% Italian; Dad was 100% Lebanese. Everybody in the family loves to cook both cuisines. Mom used to kill chickens in the basement, wash raw turkeys in the sink, and throw them on the kitchen table before cooking dinner, no thoughts of germs at ALL. And none of my brothers and sisters ever got sick, including me.

Dad was also a good cook! He taught us a lot about the traditional Lebanese dishes he grew up with, like lamb meat pies, kibbeh, tabouleh, lamb and onions and don't forget the desserts. I am very proud to say that Dad was a Purple Heart Veteran. He was a tail gunner on B52 gunners, and his plane was shot out of a tree during World War II. They told him he'd never have kids due to a missing body part accident (yes, ouch to all the men out there!), but he ended up having eight children. Me—I'm right in the middle.

Sunday dinners were legendary, and sometimes homemade pasta filled the kitchen table, hung off all the chairs and spread into the dining room to dry. Every so often, the family would gather for a day and have a "Lebanese Cook-Off," meaning we cooked lamb meat pies, spinach and feta triangle pies, tabouleh, hummus, and tahini. We cooked and ate all day long. Dave loved these family gatherings, especially since he lost his mom and dad very early in our marriage.

As a Road Warrior for over thirty years, when I was home, I cooked every single night. Early on in our marriage, Dave realized it was therapy for me! I would come home from a stressful week on the road, or a stressful day with a customer, and he'd catch me singing and dancing in the kitchen.

Cooking for Dave was a pleasure, and he was a good guy to experiment on. He'd come home from the firehouse, and I'd be in the kitchen. Dave loved my cooking and always said why go out when I have such good meals at home? If a dish was particularly good, he'd say, "This is company worthy." Amazingly, there was only one meal he didn't like over our entire time together. It was a shrimp dish with some kind of sauce, and he said, "That's just a waste of good shrimp!!" One meal out of thirty years cooking for this man was a good record.

My dedication to cooking was about more than reliving memories with Dave. It was about saving my own life as well. After Dave died, I knew I had to keep cooking because if I didn't, I'd start eating fast food and junk, and my health would decline. Cooking for one became a necessity with my new healthy lifestyle and new food plan.

It was also a constant reminder that I was alone.

Even though I can always find something fairly healthy while on the road when I was still working or traveling for pleasure, it wasn't always 100% organic, and maybe not exactly grass-fed beef or organic chicken! It was another motivation to keep cooking at home and packing my own travel snacks.

My Functional Medicine doctor, Dr. Jimerson, asked me what my flow was during one of our visits healing my rotator cuff. After I asked "Sir Google" what flow was, I came across the description of flow as kind of like a runner's high; you lose track of time, thought, and space and totally immerse yourself into an activity with tremendous focus. I realized cooking was my flow. Dave had realized way back then that it was my "flow" therapy, and it remains my passion to this day.

When I was traveling every week and eating on the road for the one year before I retired and the whole year and a half after Dave died, it certainly had its challenges. If I have a blender in a room, then I can make smoothies. If there's a fry pan, I can make grass fed burgers and sautéed greens. Salmon is always easy to make if you're in a hotel with a kitchen. I always try to find a hotel brand that has a full-service kitchen, or even an Airbnb instead of just a room with a bed. Before I leave home for the trip, I'll pack a bag with carrots, celery, cucumber, radishes, and an apple for the plane ride or car trip. I love my organic green granny smith apples. I learned some tips and tricks on the road, like packing snack bags with organic nuts, and don't forget the little packets of sea salt.

I was invited to be the "Guest Chef" at our neighborhood club. What a blast that was, both planning and prepping for this day. It gave me a sense of purpose doing something I loved with Dave, and all our friends came out that night. I had this recipe that I first made for Dave but has since been modified. It has evolved into my signature house specialty. The recipe is Champagne Chicken Thighs with organic roasted sweet potatoes and organic toasty broccoli.

Chef Mike at the club let me into his kitchen to tour around and I remember telling him, "If it's going to have my name on it, it's going to be organic, because it's that important." I bought organic avocado oil and twenty pounds of organic sweet potatoes. I helped peel them, and it reminded me of growing up and peeling those ten pounds on many nights for family sized mashed potatoes. Chef Mike found organic chicken thighs from his food vendor that he was quite excited about. And then we cooked.

The event was sold out, I helped serve everyone, and it was awesome. That night, either every single person lied, or every single person loved the meal. One guest even complained that someone else's sweet potato portion was bigger. Nothing was left on anyone's plate, and there were lots of rave reviews. I had a lot of requests for the recipe which is the highest form of compliment a cook could ever receive.

The inspiration for my next book, *Cooking with a Side of Kleenex*, came out of my health journey and my new life's purpose of helping others. Why the title for my cookbook? Well, cooking for just me made me realize there's a LOT of widows and widowers who will just say, "It's just me. I don't feel like cooking for just one" or "I can't just cook for one." If you want to stay healthy and live long and prosper, your health has to be the number one priority. And if you don't cook for yourself, it's a slippery slope, lined with fast food, sugar, unhealthy choices, and snacks, which will eventually make you feel like crap. And if you feel like crap, you won't have the energy for Life Part 2.

Cooking for that first year brought me joy, tears, and a sense of accomplishment to know I was keeping myself healthy and strong. Nutrition really is the cornerstone of health; without good food, you won't feel well or live well or even find something to laugh about. How you nourish your body is the single most essential step in healing from the inside out.

So, grab a box of Kleenex, get your apron on, and let's cook!

CHAPTER 11

A Corona Love Story

*A*s my body began to heal, so did my mind. As my mind began to heal, so did my soul. I was moving closer and closer to being open and ready for Life Part 2.

To top off the incredible month of February after graduating as a Certified Health Coach, my leader from the coaching academy, Mahnaz, asked me to speak at a Functional Medicine Coaching Academy conference she was hosting in London, England. I was wildly excited, and it was going to be the debut of my coaching future and my book launch. Believe it or not, the speech was titled "Manifesting with Velocity," a phrase that would embody what was to come next.

Sarasota is a pretty special city. I picked this place to move to after spending New Year's Eve here the year before. After my month's rental on the Siesta Key beach, I knew I was hooked. Dave and I had always thought we'd be on the Atlantic Coast of Florida, never the Gulf Coast. I explored and fell in love with the culture, restaurants, nightlife, golf, and social Meetup groups in this Florida city.

I joined a couple of Meetup groups—wine tastings, golf groups, singles groups. Then I started a Meetup group of my own called "Widowhood Sucks—Especially After 50". Other groups I joined in Sarasota included Suncoast Duffers for golfers, Girlfriends Having Dinner, and other social groups with varied interests.

Sarasota had live bands every single night of the week at many different venues, with early shows starting at 6:00 p.m. instead of later in the evening. I was in heaven. This was the city for me, and I felt it in my heart. I even bought a new dress to wear to the Sarasota Opera, knowing I might very well be going by myself. After being a solo female traveler for my whole life, it didn't bother me to go out alone. Apprehensive, yes, but I was determined to embrace life again and do things that I loved, even if it was alone.

It was about a year and a half after Dave died when I decided to entertain the possibility of dating again. At the same time, I was hoping to expand my social connections and make new friends. Michael Boyle wrote a book titled *A Friend is a Gift You Give Yourself.* How true is that? It's funny, because I've always been very outgoing, enjoyed having people around, and still had lots of love to give, and here I was, alone in a new city. Of course, my passion for cooking for others was another driver for that decision to date again. I do love to cook for others!

I was used to eating alone from my many years of travel for work. The first few times I did it as a widow, though, it felt extra strange. It made me feel awkward, like I was being stared at in an entirely uncomfortable way. Could people see I was a widow? Did I have a scarlet capital *W* on my forehead? What am I projecting? Do I look too sad?

I am thankful for the strength and perseverance I had in my bones to move away from this nagging voice in my head.

When I look back, I realize how healing myself from the inside as well as outside led to my heart opening, ready to let love in again. I eliminated the chronic stress I lived with for years, and when I got fit and slim, it boosted my confidence and self-esteem. The stress came from work, being overweight, having chronic autoimmune issues and from being a caregiver to both Dave and all his health challenges as well as helping my parents for at least fifteen years before they passed away. I finally felt good and alive!

One night I was having dinner, alone, at a wonderful restaurant in downtown Sarasota called Mattison's, with really good farm-to-table food. They featured nightly bands and dancing, and I love to dance. As I was finishing up my dinner at the bar, by myself because my friend didn't show up, I noticed this handsome guy with a huge smile on his face lighting up the room, dancing to every song with anyone available. Our eyes met, we were both smiling, and before we knew it, we were dancing, talking, and laughing together the rest of the night. This was so odd, enjoying dancing with someone else besides Dave. The first slow dance that was played that night was incredibly emotional, in a good way. In a handsome stranger's arms and smiling again—I couldn't believe it!

It affirmed my decision to go out that evening and stay to eat dinner alone. Why shouldn't I enjoy dining alone? Can you imagine if I left and didn't meet eyes and smile back at this handsome stranger? The saying "a smile begets a smile" ran through my mind—how true that is.

That night began my relationship with Jeff. I was really just looking for an adventure partner, someone to travel with, never imagining having another love like Dave's. I had no expectations at this early stage, but it was great fun having someone around who was such a joy to be with.

Jeff was in Sarasota, arriving the week before I did, working on a project in construction with a company who renovated beach resorts. His project in Sarasota ended the day I moved into my condo, about a month after we met, but he was able to be there to help me and Brooke (who helped me move out of my house and flew down to help me move in the condo) move out of the beach rental over the weekend. It was a strange feeling, I *needed* Brooke there to help me get organized, she's a pro, and at the same time, I *wanted* Jeff there! I wanted them both there, to be honest, but wasn't sure how Brooke would feel. She was just fine though and liked Jeff from the beginning, especially seeing the two of us together acting like kids.

I'll never forget the first time Jeff kissed me, and kissed me, and kissed me. It was one of those never-ending kisses, incredibly emotional and passionate. Even today, when he gets this loving look in his eyes and we kiss, the chills run up my spine, and I melt. Talk about feeling like a teenager again!

Jeff loves to eat, and I love to cook, so what a match made in heaven. He's the first man I cooked for after Dave died. That first dinner on Siesta Key at my Airbnb condo was pretty special; I felt like Dave was looking over me and smiling. Probably laughing his butt off, actually, as I sang and danced around the kitchen before Jeff arrived, just like when we were first married. I made one of my house specialties, "Marie's Seafood Boil." It had a lot of shrimp (Jeff's favorite), clams, mussels, crab legs, potatoes, and a little kielbasa. There were NO leftovers that night.

Jeff had been divorced for over ten years when we met. He was in a number of relationships over those years, and remarkably tried to learn something from each one of them to make him a better person and partner. One of his friends in the beginning told Jeff, just stop, stay by yourself, and figure out what you want in life instead of just jumping from relationship to relationship. So he did. Apparently what he was looking for was me!

I sent him the article *10 Things to Know Before Dating a Widow*, and he read every word of it. The one that stuck out for him was number ten which said that "the amount of love a widow has to offer is remarkable, so you better be ready for it." He is also very conscious and respectful of Dave and our life together, realizing that I would not be with him or be the woman I am today if it wasn't for our marriage before we met. He's right, my love and relationship with Dave was so positive and good and it forged the way for me to find another great love of the same strength. At times I felt it was too good to be true, but I knew the work I had been doing on my mind, body, and soul was what was attracting such an incredible partner.

Jeff's project in Sarasota ended in early February, and he went on to his next project in Rockland, Maine. My heart sank when I dropped him off at the airport; it was an awful feeling. He flew back to Maine and began work at a beautiful golf resort (one of the top golf resorts in the US) called Samoset. Valentine's Day was coming up, and I decided to fly up and see him. I couldn't wait to see him, actually, and it had been a whole ten days since he left Sarasota.

Remarkably, the morning I flew to Maine, the very last Valentine's Day card Dave gave to me (and the very last card ever) somehow rose to the top of the bedroom drawer as I was packing. What are the odds of that? Another Dave wink.

This was going to be just my second Valentine's Day without Dave, and the first with a new man in my life. It used to be one of our favorite holidays together, and we always celebrated every single year in many different ways. So here I am in a strange city with a man I've known for only a month, even though we were together day and night since we met. As each day went on with this wonderful man, I continued to have little nagging thoughts in my head, thoughts like *is this too good to be true? Is there something that will come slam me to the ground that's right around the corner?* Yet every time Jeff and I reconnected, all he had to do was smile at me in his loving way with those ocean blue eyes. As time went on, I knew it was going to be alright, and this was real true love again.

We ended up having a beautiful and romantic Valentine's dinner and a special evening at the Samoset resort up in Rockland, Maine. We headed to "camp" on Saturday morning, about two hours away in Franklin, near Bar Harbor, Maine. We arrived, and I remember looking around at this beautiful place, and I said, "This is not a 'camp.' This is a lake house!"

When I decided to fly up to see Jeff in Maine, one of my friends said to me, "You hardly know this man. How can you fly up alone to see him for a long weekend?" We had been inseparable since the third week in January, together every night. If we weren't together, we were on Facetime three-to-four-hours a day. I knew it was for real, and Jeff knew as well. I laugh when I think back on my friend Brooke's comment that we could not move in together until we had an argument. I'd turn to Jeff daily and say, "Are you ready? Want to fight?"

I also met Tucker the cat that weekend. There's something about a man and a cat. Of course, Tucker is a Maine Coon cat, with the loudest purr you ever heard. I learned from Sir Google that the Maine Coon cat is the largest domesticated cat breed. It has a distinctive physical appearance and valuable hunting skills, which is a good thing, because Tucker doesn't come inside very often. It is native to the state of Maine, and it's the official state cat. Tucker may be a hunter at heart, but he is also a purring teddy bear and loves to cuddle, just like Jeff. It felt good to be around the things he loved. I was learning to love them too.

I flew home from Maine, not wanting to leave and feeling lonely already. Still, I had a lot to look forward to. February was a memorable month in so many ways. One of the biggest things that happened was moving into my glorious condo overlooking Sarasota Bay, and Jeff was there to help.

Meanwhile, ten days after Valentine's Day, Jeff had a week off from the project in Rockland. And he decided to fly down to Sarasota to see me. It was a very special week; we explored the city, golfed, watched the sunsets from the balcony, went to the beach, and even went down to see what turned out to be the very last spring training game of the Boston Red Sox. It was a lovely, passionate week, and we had a great time together. We were totally comfortable with each other (even leaving the bathroom door open!). Jeff left after a week, and I still really didn't know how this was going to work out. We were so far apart, in different states, not near each other.

Maine and Florida aren't exactly a short drive—1,642 miles away to be exact.

That's when Covid decided to rear its ugly head and threw us together, unknowingly to both of us at that point.

It was a Thursday morning. I was packed and all checked in for my flight to London to speak at the Functional Medicine Coaching Academy. I had been retired from Oracle since January, so I could spend a lot of time working on my speech called "Manifesting with Velocity." It was going to be my first on stage appearance to launch my book, my new career as a Wellness Coach, and my first speaking engagement hopefully leading to more opportunities to get the word out about what I was doing in Life Part 2. I was rehearsing like crazy up to the day of departure, and then the world shut down, literally.

The night before, the order was issued about travel out of the country due to this new thing called COVID-19. I knew in my heart I could get to London no problem but getting home might be a different issue. I raised the concern in a message to Mahnaz, and she called me right back from London. Mahnaz ended up cancelling the entire event that day; there were people coming in from all over the world, and they just couldn't travel. Mahnaz actually couldn't get home to her family in Saudi Arabia for another three months!

I was sitting in my condo, thinking, *now what?* I said, "Heck, I'll just fly up and see Jeff for a week." I was going to leave that Sunday, but I remember my friend said, "Don't wait, because you might not get out. You better leave Saturday." I told her that was impossible because I had to pack and dig up some warm clothes, shut the condo down, and she said, "So? Just do it!" So, I did, packing enough for only one week and left two days later on a Saturday. Mind you, it had only been less than ten days since Jeff left, and I was missing him like crazy, again. My heart was fluttering as the plane descended into the Bangor, Maine airport. There I was, in my raincoat and snakeskin boots.

The short visit turned into two and a half months before we could get south again. Jeff picked me up at the airport in Bangor, Maine (home of the famous writer Stephen King). We had an amazing night and a dinner which turned out to be our last dinner out on the town, and Maine shut down the very next day. I couldn't get out of Maine because of COVID. I traveled with Jeff back and forth to Samoset while he worked on the resort renovations during the week. Every day was an adventure. The resort had totally shut down, no restaurants, no housekeeping, no laundry, no pool, no gym, no services, period. And no toilet paper.

Toilet paper—why did this unlikely shortage happen during the pandemic? During the early stages, there was a shortage everywhere, in stores or online. Of course, there was nothing open at the Samoset resort. Sometimes, with no rhyme or reason, the housekeeping rooms would be open at the resort, they'd get a fresh delivery of supplies, and we'd go raiding the cupboards. Jeff has pictures of me with rolls of toilet paper under my sweatshirt laughing hysterically as we emptied out in the room! Thieves in the night. I'm sure we're on video somewhere, and it will come back to haunt us when we're ninety.

We made an adventure of it and laughed about so many things. Every day, in the electric skillet, I would cook breakfast for Jeff, he'd go off to work, and I'd do dishes in the bathroom tub. Jeff would come home for lunch, and I'd cook deer burgers or moose steaks on the skillet. There was one grocery store still open about a mile away, and that would be my daily exercise, shopping for fresh organic vegetables and seafood for dinner. We learned a lot about each other, and we became very at ease and comfortable with the relationship, as if we'd been together for years. I also learned that Jeff loved Oreos or chocolate with almond milk after each meal. I am so happy to report that not one single Oreo passed my lips, and I hope to continue that streak forever. Doing dishes in the bathtub was a riot, AND we had to do our own laundry and cleanup. We'd leave for camp on Friday nights and stay there until Sunday when we returned to the resort. Rinse and repeat! Even though Jeff and Dave were completely different in their ways, habits, and communication styles, both relationships were connected with a common theme of laughter and love.

Each weekend, we'd head back to Jeff's place at Abrams Pond, and each week that passed I turned into a Walmart shopper and a Carhartt girl (to Jeff's delight!). It's actually pronounced "Cah-haht." here in Maine. They are known for their rugged work and hunting clothes. I remember talking with my friend Cyndy about my new shopping trips, and she would say, "Excuse me, have you seen my friend Marie?" I was simultaneously transforming, while also feeling more like my old self, as I settled into camp life in remote Maine. I was coming back to life.

I shared pictures on social media of me in Carhartt pants, camo vests, and big boots (in Jeff's boots at first, until I found my own). I managed to buy the very last parka at Walmart, two sizes too big, but I was desperate. I wore that coat the whole winter, and I was thankful for how warm it kept me.

One day in April, a Wednesday to be exact, Jeff said, "Pack up. We're leaving Samoset!" Some of the crew he was working with were not well, probably COVID, and he was not feeling safe. I said "*What?!*" I packed up our room, which had a TON of stuff in it, like skillets, dishes, a refrigerator full of food and dry goods on all the shelves. Not to mention our precious stash of toilet paper rolls. We headed to camp and decided to start work on construction of two more bedrooms and a big garage. This had been Jeff's dream for a very long time, and COVID just made it happen.

We laid the foundation for the 24x40' garage, and we etched into a corner of the concrete "Jeff and Marie, a Corona Love Story." In the opposite corner, where the bathroom was, Jeff etched "Dad's Throne" as a funny tribute to his father.

Construction was a welcome diversion. During the days, I was working on launching my wellness business, courses, website, and finishing the book, while Jeff worked outside from sunrise to sunset. I helped him a lot too, and I think I made a good apprentice. He taught me how to use a bunch of power tools and bought me my own palm hammer. I even got to use the electric chainsaw helping him cut some trees down. He's a really good teacher with lots of patience.

So, because of COVID, we thrived, and it brought us closer together. It truly was the best quarantine ever. We're thankful every single day for our good fortune in meeting. Jeff turned out to be another fellow adventurer, loves to travel, and is spontaneous like me. He's passionate, smart, funny, considerate, thoughtful, kind, and sensitive. Not to mention a great dancer, and he loves to golf. Jeff loves to hear about my travels with Dave, so conscious of how much history we made over our time together and loved stories about our successful relationship. He looks forward to revisiting some of the same places, like Toronto, Charleston, Vancouver, and overseas. Jeff is so good about honoring my old memories while making new ones of our own.

I look back on the winter in Maine and it reminds me of my first awesome winter with Dave when he said, "Quit your job! Come to Canada! Come skiing!" Well, the winter in Maine was just as awesome. Can a person have two best winters in their life? I say yes, as it was happening to me. Here I was, healing inside and out, and falling in love again, head over heels. Winters lead to spring, my favorite time of year, and this love was blossoming fiercely, just as it had with Dave.

We laugh and giggle and smile every single day, like we're twenty-nine years old. From the minute we wake up, even if it's in the middle of the night, we make each other smile, and it's an incredible feeling. The passion and excitement for life is so apparent and obvious coming from us both, that everyone in our circle of family and friends can see and embrace how happy we are. Two peas in a pod.

How crazy was this—finding a second great love in my life.

Jeff said the "F" word first, the *forever* word, only two months after we started dating.

When he said it, I was left speechless (very unusual).

"*Forever*." How could he say this! And I remember saying to him, "How can you know!"

He said to me, holding his fist to his chest, "I feel it in my heart."

He let me reorganize his kitchen during quarantine, and that's when I said to him, "You realize we just moved in with each other, don't you?" Just like teenagers, and now we're "shacking up!" We never did have that first fight like Brooke said we had to before moving in together—lots of laughs but no fights. It was surreal being with this wonderful man, looking and waiting for the first argument, the first fight, the first disagreement. There weren't any. You know what? If and when that does happen, our love is so strong, we're so mature, and the communication between us is so good, that I know we're ready to overcome that first fight, so bring it on!

Jeff had a motorhome which he was going to sell. As time went on, week after week with no end in sight to the state borders opening up, I said, "You might want to keep the motor home. It may be the only way I ever get home to Florida." And it turned out to be true.

What an adventure the trip down south was, my first in a motorhome. My idea of camping my whole life was a Hilton and room service. In retrospect, I call it the "Meet the Family Tour." We started out with an oil change for the motorhome in Bangor, then headed south to meet his mom in Brunswick, Maine, for a late lunch. I was nervous! It had been a very long time—at least forty years— since I was in a position to meet the parents of a new man I was dating for the first time. Mom Joyce is a beautiful soul. She made me instantly comfortable and at ease. Her spirit shined bright, and I could tell this is where Jeff got his good looks and smile from. She had an instant curiosity of how this new woman in his life was treating her only son! She could also tell how tired Jeff looked, since it had been an intense week leading up to this departure from Maine after being there for almost three months.

It had been a very long day. We got back in the Motorhome and drove for about five hours. We ended up at a truck stop in Charlton, Massachusetts. I made my sister Kathy laugh the next day with this story. My dad was a long-distance truck driver, coast to coast, when we were growing up. And I swear I saw my dad at that truck stop that night in my dreams! Heck of a way to start my first adventure in a motorhome, parked among the big rigs. It got better after that; we had a great adventure in Rochester to meet my family. We parked the motor home in brother Mike's driveway and had three great days of golf, dinners, and meeting my (large) family, and they all loved Jeff. Next up was Virginia Beach just so we could have some more fun, and then Summerville, South Carolina, to meet my dear friends and old neighbors. They approved of Jeff and best of all could see how happy I was, how happy and comfortable we both were. There wasn't one moment of feeling awkward, or unsure of how people who knew Dave would react, especially my family.

We took the motorhome back to Maine in July to continue construction. Back at camp my brothers and nephew drove up from Rochester to help us get ready for "hunting season," whatever that was. I just didn't know yet what was in store for that week (or two!). My brothers and nephew Greg are so talented. Brother Mike is the all-around inside remodeler. Brother Rich is the lifelong mason while nephew Greg is the world's best framer of houses. They all drove up together, bringing their favorite tools of their trades. Sister-in-law Cindy drove up separately, and it was great having her with me with all the action going on. That week, we got the addition framed and the roof put on. Major accomplishment, and it wasn't all work; there was golfing, fishing, fine dining, and cooking all week. It was so good to blend our families together.

My brother said to me during one of our alone moments, "We liked the golf course where you and Dave lived because we love to golf, but that's all there was. Here, it's beautiful. The lake was waiting every night to go fishing. There's fresh air, and we still golf!" He also commented on how "adaptable" I was, going from Sarasota city life to country life in Maine. High heels to mud boots.

My brother Rich the mason built a pink granite wall facade in front with stones Jeff gathered from a tree project (my very own Paul Bunyan, his career was in forestry) he had completed near the ocean in Bar Harbor, Maine. Jeff has a heart rock which he has treasured, tucked in a special spot down by the beach at camp.

Rich just happened to find another heart rock while he was taking a leak on the property next door, and that is now the centerpiece

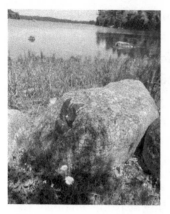

of the wall. The jury is out whether he actually peed on the heart rock or just near it! I don't want to know.

Hearts are definitely a sign for us, with more to come. In fact, Jeff's mom, Mom Joyce as I call her, gave us a special heart rock which will be a centerpiece of the next wall we build outside.

Jeff had cousins. I had no idea of quite how many there were though. I heard about this event called "Pie Week" and had no idea what that meant either. Turned out it was a family reunion which had been held for years and years. It started on Friday night with cousins Cheryl and Heidi banging at our door in a panic, yelling about tornado warnings! They had just set up their camper that night and ended up closing it down and headed to our place. We were just arriving after having driven back from a whole day near the coast, golfing and having a fine lobster dinner, so we were tired and not ready for what was about to happen.

Well, the roof had other ideas. It wasn't watertight yet. All of a sudden, I noticed rain pouring down the living room wall coming from the roof. The guys rallied, trying to figure out what to do. My nephew Greg, like Spiderman, climbed up on the roof. With the howling winds and torrential rain, he had arms and legs out over the peak trying to hold the tarp down while the guys tried to get it stapled down. Greg, I still owe you a pair of golf pants for the ones that got ruined that night.

So that's how Pie Week started, and my introduction began to the numerous cousins. I joked with Jeff that he had to draw me a chart of the family tree, and with his mom, we did come up with a wonderful family chart which helped me a lot to figure out who was who. As the weekend neared, more arrived and set up camps all around Abrams Pond, and the whole group went from campfire to campfire, laughing, playing games, and hoisting a few adult beverages.

It was so comforting to me to be around such good people, all of them very close, and their love for Jeff was obvious. His laugh is infectious, his smile lights up the room, and his love for me is so affectionate and passionate it feels really good. They saw both of us embarking on a journey of finding love again in a real lasting way. What a good match for both of us.

Sunday was the culmination of the week, called "Pie Sunday." Just as the name implied, there were a LOT of pies, I think at least thirty homemade pies, along with a great cookout. That morning, tradition was for all able bodies to swim to the "island" in the middle of Abrams Pond. I am not a particularly strong swimmer (plus I'm a chicken when it comes to bodies of water larger than my bathtub), so I volunteered to row alongside the swimmers as a "spotter." It was an awesome week of fun, campfires, games on the lawn, and good food.

My first Maine lobster feast was with Jeff, and I always joked about who had the better lobster—Maine or Nova Scotia. I spent many years on projects in Nova Scotia and loved the sweetness of their lobsters. I will admit (don't tell Jeff) that Maine lobster, fresh off the boat, is amazing. He has this large pot which holds twenty-five–thirty lobsters at least, cooked for exactly twenty-two minutes. The first time I went shopping for lobster, Jeff asked me, "How many are you getting?" A little surprised, I said, "One for each of us?" Wrong answer! Come to find out the minimum number was at least three for Jeff. He likes nothing on it, just pure lobsters picked clean. The leftovers, if there were any, went to making lobster rolls, and mine were pretty popular. Just a little mayo, grilled buttered rolls, and maybe a touch of celery. That's it!

Meeting his dad for the first time was great. His contagious smile and laugh reminded me of Jeff! He also has a full head of beautiful hair, just like Jeff. Jeff told me Dad loved to eat (just like him!) and with my love of cooking, it was another great match. I learned how to cook deer meat lasagna, deer meat chili, moose meat bourguignon, and these all became favorites of both the guys.

Ever since I met Jeff, he talked with reverence about this thing called "hunting week." With my love of cooking and his love of hunting, he had visions of us resurrecting the tradition of everyone being together, sleeping and hunting right here at camp. It would be just like growing up with his dad and mom and the hunters. Not knowing what this meant, I dove in with both feet. We were just finishing the two-bedroom addition that Friday. The furniture just got delivered, and we washed the new linens and made the beds, and voila! The hunters started arriving from all over the northeast. These were long time connections for many years. Wayne from upstate New York was first on Thursday; he'd been coming up to "camp" for at least fifty years. Tippy and his son Bobby from Connecticut had been coming up hunting for sixty years! Dad Gordon showed up and stayed with us until the deer meat was processed the following Sunday. Cousins Mike and Bill, and Christopher and Ralph, rounded out the week. A special group of men, all very close and all so passionate about this one week a year—hunting week.

Boy, did I have a blast. Every morning, the guys would rise at 4:00 a.m., and as I lay in bed, I could hear them all talking deer hunting strategy—who was going where and when. They'd all go out before sunrise, and I'd get up, ready to feed them at noon. My macaroni salad was a big hit, along with lobster rolls, sweet potatoes, ribs, chicken, and deer meat chili. We went to town (not close at all) a couple of times, which was a nice break for the chief cook and bottlewasher (me). Cooking, cleaning, and laundry every day was the theme song in my head. When the guys were done and returned to camp, I loved hearing the stories of the day and the days past. The deer sizes grew bigger as the campfire blazed and the cigars were lit.

Maine hunting rules are you can go out a half an hour before sunrise and be in a half an hour after sunset. One of Jeff's wishes for the new garage with its "game" room, or deer office, was that dad have the honor of the first deer hanging. Dad Gordon is a wonderful man. Jeff and he are very close, and I love listening to their conversations. Dad's laugh is as infectious as Jeff's. I immediately felt close to him.

It could have been because I like to cook and he likes to eat, but I imagine it's because he loved me too and appreciated the happiness I brought to his son.

I went out with Jeff on a hike during the start of hunting week, and we ended up in one of his garden hunting plots where we sat quietly in one of the tree houses as sunset fast approached. We sat scanning the fields for deer. All of a sudden, we heard a BOOM, just one shot, and Jeff knew immediately what it was. He smiled and turned to me and said, "That's Dad." Dad was sitting in his tree shack (we call it the "love shack") next door. I asked Jeff, "Is Dad Gordon a good shot?" and he replied back, "Heck yeah!" We went over to where the shot came from and hooked up with dad. Then he and Jeff went tracking the deer. I was happy this dream came true for Jeff—having Dad's deer hanging in the garage first. That hunting week, the guys shot five bucks, the biggest being 194 pounds by Cousin Bill. I never did go near the garage, because I can't stand the sight of blood, and Jeff understands that about me. I'll cook it happily, just don't make me look at it!

I was still trying to finish my book, work on my website, and had weekly calls with team members and coaches like Thomas and Whitney during the week. I warned them that if they saw a bunch of guys walking in with rifles slung on their shoulders, don't be alarmed. I wasn't in danger—it's only the hunters! Of course, it did happen and was just one more thing to laugh about.

Thanksgiving dinner was special, at a wonderful place called the Lucerne Inn. It was special because it had been many years since I looked forward to the holidays. The year Dave was diagnosed happened around Thanksgiving, and that was the last time I enjoyed this time of year. It was odd being happy at dinner, and I felt weird until I started quieting the negative self-talk in my head and gave myself permission to be happy. As Christmas approached, I was ready to decorate again, the first time in years!

Once hunting week season was over in Maine, we were ready to head south. We packed up the motorhome and hit the road pointed straight south. We usually took our time and planned adventures, but it was cold on our trip south, and we wanted to get warm fast. I did buy a small Charlie Brown Christmas tree and a cute Troll we nicknamed Nick and we decorated the condo in Florida for Christmas. It was the first time I felt like having decorations up, the first time since Dave's brain aneurysm about ten years before. It was lovely having his sister Brenda and Aunt Sybil join us for a couple of nights, and it made the Christmas holiday so warm and wonderful.

The morning of our one-year anniversary, we had a golf tee time set for a Disney course in Orlando. I set the alarm, and when it went off early that morning, the ring tone was this:

"Honey pick up, hey, hello, it's your husband. Hello, pick up, Honey, seriously, I need to talk to you, what are you doing?"

Jeff lying beside me chuckled and just thought it was Dave's voice recorded (it wasn't) as one of my ringtones. I was shocked this purchased ringtone from years and years ago was still around waiting to pop up! I look back now and I think it was Dave giving his okay and support to go ahead—maybe another God wink for what would happen next.

That night, he really got me. Jeff totally surprised and shocked me on our one-year anniversary by asking me to marry him, on a Zoom call with family and friends. I thought he just wanted a happy hour anniversary cheers-to-us party! He turned to me and said, "Will you marry me?" The tears started flowing, and I couldn't believe my ears, speechless once again since he said the "F" word a year before! He put the ring on my finger (it fit perfectly, of course) and after about a minute someone yelled, "So, did she say yes!?" I did say yes, over and over. He took this beautiful ring off his necklace and placed it on my hand with me thinking, *how could this be happening? My heart may just burst!* The ring is one of a kind, it is heart shaped (more hearts to add to our story) which he designed. It's got both our birthstones in it, sapphire and aquamarine with a diamond in the middle. Etched inside the ring is: "A Corona Love Story."

Jeff wants me to keep Scott as my middle name, as a tribute to Dave. He's been so remarkable about treasuring the memories and stories and travels I share with him about Dave and our past life together. Besides, I kind of like the sound of *Marie Scott Gordon*, even as it chokes me up thinking about my happiness with this man and my happiness with Dave. How can it be possible to have two great loves in one lifetime? I am one lucky girl.

Someone asked me recently if it was awkward for my family (and Jeff's) to see us with other people. The answer is a resounding NO.—nothing awkward at all about our friends or family feeling ecstatic that we have found each other. Jeff's mom and sister talk about how we have such a "harmony" together, and we do. We talk about what it would have been like if we had met twenty years ago, and we both agree it wouldn't have worked. We are both in the right time and place for this to have happened when it did.

We are building a new life together, with great plans for many adventures for the rest of our lives, hoping to live to at least one hundred. It's funny being part of a couple again, doing things together, doing life together, and talking about the future. When this part of me came to a screeching halt when Dave died, I never dreamed it would come back as strongly as it has. I am grateful it has become a welcome and beautiful part of my life.

For our first Valentine's Day, I bought Jeff a card in the shape of a heart, and he still keeps it on his pillow if I'm not there. I love his sentimentality.

Writing this book has been a wonderful experience. I kept a file of "Miscellaneous Book Notes" and recently went back through to make little additions from the napkins, Post-it Notes, notepad notes, cardboard coasters, and anything else I could find to write on at the time a thought came across my mind. It's a very colorful file!

One note in particular stopped me in my tracks. I was creating a vision board for life and the book, about a year and a half after Dave died. I found a note called "Love Partner." This couldn't have described Jeff better. Fit, Funny, Vibrant, Sexy, Affectionate, Healthy and Kind. Oh—and did I mention—a great dancer who loves to golf? Jeff and I haven't stopped dancing since that first time.

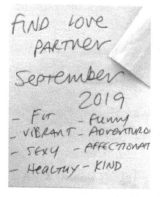

Most widows I have met and interacted with have no desire to have another man in their life. I wasn't looking to get married again either; it wasn't in my plans or thoughts at all. Some of the comments and posts I've read in my widow groups are: "I've had the best; forget the rest" or "I'll never date again; he was my one and only." Seriously, that's what I thought too until I began to heal myself all the way around. In the weirdest year ever at a time when the world shut down and we were separated from everyone and everything "normal", the world sent me Jeff.

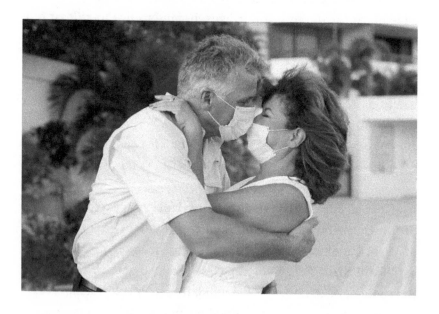

This is a true "Corona Love Story" and a great way to spend the rest of my life, "Life Part 2."

Live well, Laugh more, Love again—Life Part 2—
I am Living Proof it is possible!

CHAPTER 12

The Shadow You Cast

I spent thirty years in technology in many different roles, mostly with Oracle. When I was a sales consultant, our Vice President and one of the most exemplary leaders I ever met and worked for, was Russell Pike. He always stressed in his closing statements during our monthly team calls, "Be aware of the shadow you cast."

Russell told me the phrase "The shadow you cast" came to his attention when he saw the Alcoa CIO (Kevin Horner) speak. He made a couple of remarks, the shadow you cast being one of them. It is truly amazing how some things just kind of stick. Russell said he's looked around a lot since then but never been able to find it specifically referred to in any formal text. It has stuck with me for all these years and now I know why it resurfaced at this time.

Here's an excerpt from Russell's blog that he wrote:

> "The **SHADOW** we cast. From the moment we get up, to the moment we go to bed, our actions, words, attitudes, and interactions impact others—that's the **SHADOW** we cast. It happens whether we like it or not, every second of the day, in everything we do; conversations, emails, tweets, status updates, blogs, even the look in our eyes and the way we carry ourselves—all are part of the **SHADOW** we cast."

Russell's blog continues with this:

*"The question is this. What is the **SHADOW** you cast? If a third party anonymously surveyed the people around you for words that describe you, what would they come back with? How does your real **SHADOW** compare to the one in your head? How would the words of those close to you compare to those on the "third" degree? Does the **SHADOW** you are actually casting reflect the person you want to be? A sobering thought in many cases."*

I never really felt the impact of this statement until Dave was gone and the stories came to light about Dave and the shadow HE cast on so many. I never realized just how much Dave impacted others until the stories were told to me after he died. Chief Al Hills said there was a story being told about Dave every day.

Dave's fellow rover scouts and oldest friends, Larry and Bob, had fond memories of Dave and the shadow he cast. Dave was an inspiration to them to be adventurers. They told me these stories about Dave which I had never heard before.

It started back when they were mere teens when they saw Dave emerge as a leader. The "Hunter's Stew" story involved the Rover crew, and the story began when they were camping and the throw down challenge was to cook dinner for the group. Their assignment was to cook beef stew with vegetables. There were two parts to the challenge. First, how good the food was, as judged by the leaders. Second, the meal had to be cooked over an open fire that had to be started without matches if possible. With Dave in the lead, the team had practiced fire starting before, using a stick to rotate quickly in a very dry log with a bit of fine wood shavings (just like as seen on TV!). The spinning stick would heat up and the friction would ignite the wood and away they went. As luck would have it, they were unsuccessful the day of the stew challenge and had to use one of the two matches they had been given as back-up by the leaders.

That was a fail on part one of the challenge, and Dave wasn't happy. There was still a chance they could win the challenge though, as Dave was usually an excellent cook. When it was ready, the leader came by for the judging. Bob can't remember why they didn't taste test the stew before the leader came to taste and judge. The leader took one spoonful and spit it out with a lot of drama. He was almost sick. They couldn't figure out what happened. It was an overload of pepper! How did it get in the stew? Maybe they were sabotaged by another crew? Bob said, "You can imagine how well Dave took the defeat. Not well." Hot dogs were for supper that night, not the stew that Dave made.

Chief Al Hills, at the memorial golf tournament, talked about how all of Dave's men rose up to be Captains. Al rose up to be Platoon Chief and says Dave had a big part in his career progression. Chief Al often talked about the great influence Dave had on his career, from rookie at the department to rising to Platoon Chief.

His best friend and fellow rover scout, Larry, came down for Dave's first annual golf memorial tournament. Dave wasn't afraid to challenge himself or others, just like he did with me our entire life together. To honor Dave's sense of adventure since they were kids and fellow scouts, Larry rode his motorcycle about seventeen hours down to South Carolina from Milton, Ontario. He said that's what Dave would do, make an adventure out of it.

We set up the annual golf memorial to benefit youth hockey scholarships, which was a love of ours. Hockey was something we both enjoyed, whether it was rooting for the South Carolina Stingrays, or helping and rooting for the Toronto Maple Leafs to get at least into the playoffs! Our memorial ended up being the biggest fundraiser for the Charleston Youth Hockey scholarships, which we will continue doing.

Dave went to the dentist every six months without fail. That didn't stop after his cancer diagnosis. When he shared the story of what was going on with him, the beautiful hygienist wrote a lovely letter to Dave the week after about how inspiring he was to her. She enclosed a copy of the poem *If* by Rudyard Kipling. The poem is about helping deal with different and difficult times in life. "*If you can keep your head when all about you Are losing theirs and blaming it on you; If you can trust yourself when all men doubt you.*"

Above all, it's how to be a good human being. I kept the letter, along with the memorable poem.

Dave, the shadow you cast continues to amaze me and brings me to tears every time with the telling of every single story from those who knew you. Lu from the YMCA told me about how intimidated you made her when you first met in 2009. You were so gruff, very forward, and brash about your issues with your knees and hips. She then came to realize how smart you were, and how determined you were to have things your own way in your healing, not to mention how stubborn you were. She told me you changed her life learning how to deal with you and your strong personality. Dave loved Lu at the Y. Loved talking to her and loved getting her opinion on his many physical challenges.

Dave's son at our last dinner told him, "Thanks, Dad, for being such a good coach in my life," and that brought a tear to Dave's eye. I heard these wise words once: you are a memory to someone, and you carry a life in this earthly body.

Peter Weiler had some awesome stories about the impact Dave had on his skiing career. We met up in Denver one time, both there on work, but we always made time for skiing. Dave was with me on one trip when we connected with Peter on the ski hill. Dave was a really good skier and a good instructor as well. Peter will never forget Dave's ski advice to, "Pretend you're carrying a TV in front of you with both hands. Keep those hands in front of you at all times!" He went on to become a member of the Canadian Ski Patrol because of Dave. He got some good advice from Dave all through his certification process, and he never forgot the TV. Peter couldn't wait to share this story with me about the shadow Dave cast on him, his skiing years, and serving on the ski patrol. It was beautiful to hear stories about how he impacted so many lives he touched.

The shadow Dave cast appeared again with a story out of Bermuda. Dave had met the now Fire Chief of Bermuda, Vince, in Gravenhurst at Fire College. Dave taught this man from Bermuda how to ski, a man who had never even seen snow before. We cruised and docked in Bermuda one year, and Dave was on a mission to find the firehouse and find this gentleman that he met thirty-five years before. Well, we did find the firehouse, and the Fire Chief just happened to be on duty that day. We sat around waiting in the kitchen, had a coffee (there was ALWAYS coffee on at the firehouse), and waited for Vince to come out of his meeting. When the Chief came out, he gave Dave the biggest hug in the world, just like it had been yesterday when they last saw each other. He then proceeded to take us on a private tour in his car around the whole island, telling many stories, and finally ended up dropping us off at our ship at the end of the day. What a beautiful experience after all those years of no contact. The Shadow You Cast lasts forever.

The Shadow I cast started in my consulting days with Oracle. One customer, the Billy Graham Organization who I helped go live with their new payroll system, asked the manager, "Where did you find Marie?" The response was, "I didn't find her. God did!" I had many happy customers who remember me fondly for the work I did. I love helping people and making them smile at the same time. One of my favorite lines to keep everyone smiling at the beginning of every week was, "Today's Monday. No whining!" Everyone can make a big difference in this world, a smile alone can change someone's day, and who knows the ripple effect that you might have on the world!

I'm the only one out of eight brothers and sisters that did not choose parenthood. My role in life was to be an aunt, and I hope I've been a good one. My niece sent me this plaque that said, "Aunts are like Moms, only Cooler!" There are so many nieces, nephews, great nieces, and great nephews that I've lost count. Dave and I had a pregnancy scare early on in our marriage, to his delight, and he had dreams of raising an Olympic skiing champion. His first thought was, *who'd quit their job though?* He was adamant one of us would be home full-time up until at least high school years. It was just a scare, thankfully, after Dave decided he'd leave his career to stay home. I do like being an aunt better than a mother. My career had me on the road a lot, so having children would not be fair if I wasn't there.

One of my favorite stories about the shadow you cast (as an aunt!) is a story with a character named Flat Stanley. One day back in 2005 I received this envelope addressed to Aunt Marie, with a flat cutout figure of "Flat Stanley." There was no indication of who it was from, just the school address. After a couple of days of detective work, I found out it was from my nephew Mike. He was probably about eight years old. My instructions were simple: take the flat guy on my adventures! At the time, I was traveling quite extensively for work, all over the US and Canada. Flat Stanley and I hit the road, from the Curling Championships in Halifax, Nova Scotia, with us on vacation in Hawaii, to work projects in Wisconsin and Chicago. I kept a journal with tidbits about each city (like cheese curds in Wisconsin!) and how far it was from home. Each city I visited, a pin was bought and attached to a wool hat. My neighbor's son crafted a couple of outfits for Stanley, including this one for #12, the quarterback for the South Carolina Gamecocks football team, which he wore to the game with 80,000 of his closest friends.

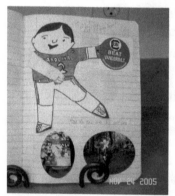

The Flat Stanley Project was originally conceived by third grade teacher Dale Hubert in Ontario Canada back in the '90s. I heard it's one of the longest-lasting literacy projects because of the simplicity of the concept. Kids send a flat visitor to someone they know, or even a celebrity or a stranger, with instructions and a timeframe. I had three months to return the flat guy to my nephew.

A package was carefully put together by Dave and me, and we sent it back to my nephew Mike. It had the hat with the pins on it, the journal, and a few other souvenirs in the box like a Wisconsin cheese head, a Lei from Hawaii, and postcards. I still have the original Flat Stanley, and I wrote a paper on my experience for my college writing course.

Mike graduated a few years back, and that's when I found out this box traveled with him wherever he moved; he kept it after all these years. What a wonderful feeling to know you've touched someone's life.

One of my favorite lines in *Hamilton* is this: "Who lives, who dies, who tells your story?" This is our story, Dave, and I'm telling it. This book motivates me to make sure I leave a legacy for us both. I hope this book is an inspiration to others who might be ready to embrace life again.

The world is a better place for Dave having lived in this lifetime. I want to make sure the world is a better place because of me living in this lifetime. I want to live a life of purpose, gratitude, and kindness, to see what kind of shadow I can cast on the world.

Life is not about just you. It's about everyone you touch.

CPSIA information can be obtained
at www.ICGtesting.com
Printed in the USA
LVHW021217251121
704321LV00002B/200